OVERCOMING TUESDAY

JIM BURNEKA JR.

HILARY HAWKINS

FOREWORD BY PATRICK J. KENNY

For information or to contact the authors follow the Link or QR Code Below

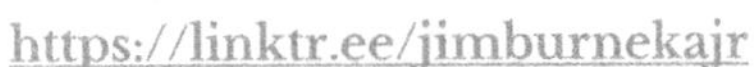

https://linktr.ee/jimburnekajr

https://linktr.ee/hilaryhawkins

ISBN: 979-8-3302-0271-3

Editor: Emily Junker

First Edition: May 2024

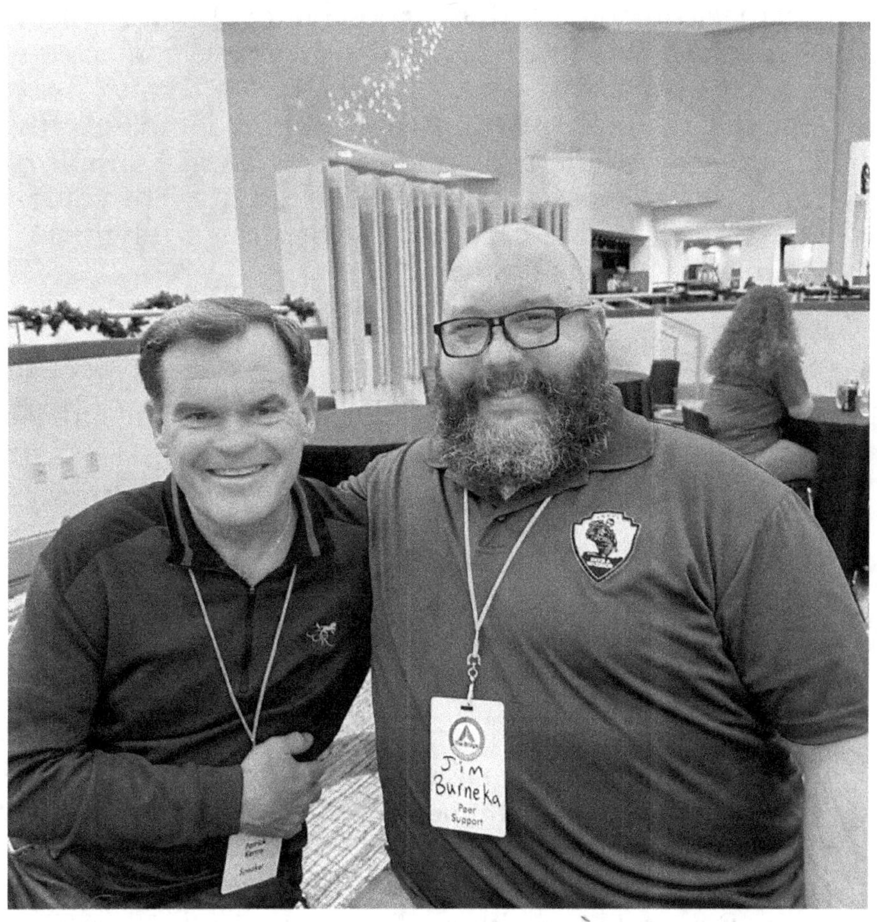

Pat Kenny and myself at the First Responders Bridge Retreat in December 2023

FOREWORD BY PATRICK J. KENNY

FIRE CHIEF (RET.)

So why did the author of *Overcoming Tuesday* select me to write this foreword? Let me give you a little history to provide the background of our relationship. I first became acquainted with my good buddy, Jim Burneka Jr., when in 2021, another friend, Dan DeGryse, contacted me about speaking with Jim at a conference in "exotic" Beavercreek, Ohio. If you think that location doesn't exactly scream "exotic," then you're witnessing a small sample of Jim's genuine sense of humor and creativity. The conference aimed to bring in speakers promoting firefighter health and wellness nationwide.

Dan was a Chicago Fire Department Battalion Chief with over thirty years of experience and had multiple certifications in the field of addiction and mental health. He also operated as the Coordinator of the Chicago Firefighters Union Local 2's Employee Assistance Program.

I was a Fire Chief at the Western Springs Fire Department in Western Springs, Illinois, with thirty-eight years of fire service experience and a Bachelor's degree in psychology. My experience with mental health was with our son, Sean, who suffered from several mental health challenges throughout his life, culminating with his death by suicide at age twenty in 2006. Starting in 2009, I began to travel the country giving lectures on mental health to first responders.

Dan and I were both a little intrigued by this conference's description, so we scheduled a video call to interview Jim. What we experienced on that call was a warm and funny man who exuded passion and sincerity in his mission to address cancer prevention and mental health awareness in the fire service. Needless to say, off we went, leading to ongoing mutual respect and friendship.

Since then, Jim has been kind enough to invite me to appear on two different podcasts—one for Fire Engineering APS radio in 2022, and then in 2023 at the Fire Department Instructor's Conference (FDIC), where I shared the stage with Dr. Sara Jahnke, director of the Center for Fire, Rescue, and EMS Health Research at the National Development and Research Institutes. Dr. Sara is one of the most respected researchers on firefighter health worldwide. You see, Jim seeks out experts in the field of firefighter wellness and then uses his charm to befriend them. I was only along to be the eye candy! That particular podcast was more like a *Saturday Night Live* skit than a training forum. Sara and I just followed Jim's lead, providing an opportunity for people to witness Jim's spontaneity and humor while still delivering firefighter safety messages.

Over the last three years, Jim and I have spoken often about the trials and tribulations of the vocation we share as firefighters. During that time, Jim supported me when I published a book, and in some of my personal challenges as I entered the retiree club. He also shared with me his own struggles in various arenas with courageous transparency. However, until I read this book, I only had a small glimpse of his suffering.

One day, he told me, "Somebody said I should write a book." I wholeheartedly endorsed the idea, as Jim has suffered through more than enough difficult experiences and has learned valuable lessons worth sharing. Little did I know he *would* write a book and turn around and ask me to write this foreword!

Why You Want To Read This Book

That brings us to this book, *Overcoming Tuesday*. You'll find a man on a journey through a difficult childhood, entering a beloved career, marrying the love of his life, having a wonderful family together, and embarking on a career dedicated to his personnels' safety. He held many roles dedicated to cancer prevention and mental health at the local and national levels. Although he had many successes in those roles, he also had major setbacks.

In this book, Jim shares with you what those journeys looked like and their associated pain, some of which could be anticipated and some which blindsided him. More importantly, he shares with you what he learned in hopes that someone going through a similar journey—not only a firefighter but any person, regardless of vocation—may be able to avoid the same struggles.

What I Love About This Book

When I read this book, I noted that Jim put a quote at the beginning of each chapter. As you read this book, I encourage you to read each quote a few times before diving into the chapter. It will help you look for key lessons learned that you might miss.

That format immediately reminded me of two people I want to quote in this foreword. The first is Theodore Roosevelt, from his famous speech about "The Man in the Arena."

"It is not the critic who counts; not the man who points out how the strong man stumbles, or where the doer of deeds could have done them better. The credit belongs to the man who is actually in the arena, whose face is marred by dust and sweat and blood; who strives valiantly; who errs, who comes short again and again, because there is no effort without error and shortcoming; but who does actually strive to do the deeds; who knows great enthusiasms, the great devotions; who spends himself in a worthy cause; who at the best knows in the end the triumph of high achievement, and who at the worst, if he fails, at least fails while daring greatly, so that his place shall never be with those cold and timid souls who neither know victory nor defeat."

Jim Burneka Jr. has been the man in the arena. He speaks of his own experiences with post-traumatic stress

disorder, organizational betrayal, cancer, and mental illness. He shares his efforts, struggles, victories, defeats, and
lessons learned. Firefighters are a breed very proud of
their strength of character, but they struggle with their
vulnerability. What Jim shares in this book is the powerful
message that vulnerability is not a weakness, but a
strength.

The book is a very easy read, but don't let that fool
you; it is full of important lessons to absorb and apply to
your life. Then, share what you've learned with people going through troubled times similar to those Jim outlines in
this book.

Finally, I would like to share the second quote I felt
compelled to use because it captures what Jim put on paper in this book. It is from the late basketball coach, Jim
Valvano, in his famous ESPY Awards speech in 1993.

*"To me, there are three things we all should do every day. . . .
Number one is laugh. You should laugh every day. Number two is
think, you should spend some time in thought. And number three
is you should have your emotions moved to tears. Could be happiness or joy, but think about it. If you laugh, you think, and you
cry, that's a full day. That's a heck of a day. You do that seven
days a week, you're going to have something special."*

When you've finished *Overcoming Tuesday,* you'll in-
deed have laughed and been brought to tears, and it will
certainly make you think. Ultimately, it will provide inval-
uable knowledge to give you hope to overcome your own
Tuesday!

Patrick J. Kenny - Keynote Speaker Mental Health Awareness and Author of the International Bestseller *Taking The
Cape Off*

CONTENTS

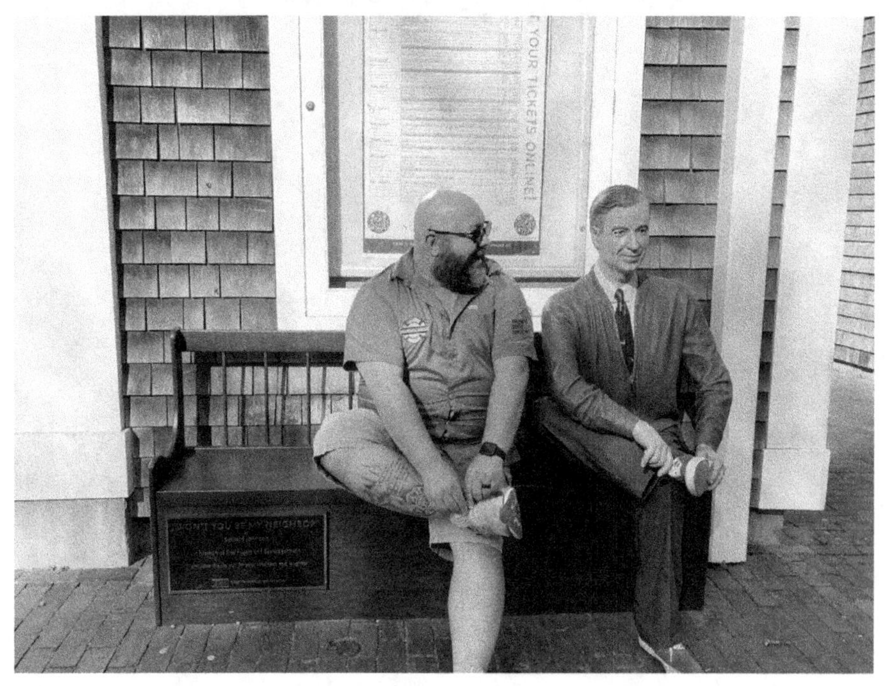

OVERCOMING
TUESDAY

1 - INTRODUCTION

*"If there's a book that you want to read, but it hasn't been written
yet, then you must write it."*
-Toni Morrison

My heart felt as though it was going to beat out of my chest. My breath was shallow as I tried to evenly speak into the microphone. I moved my hands as I spoke, hoping the tiny droplets of sweat on my palms weren't visible. The camera's bright light left me feeling exposed, as if it was illuminating the truth I was hiding. I was waiting for a producer to yell "cut" and tell me that they needed someone who was not a hypocrite—anyone but me.

If the camera had an x-ray lens, it would reveal the truth. Everyone would be able to see my bones that had been crushed by the weight of the world I was carrying. It would display my shattered heart, the fragments floating throughout my body, a constant reminder that I was not okay.

Luckily for me, it was just a regular camera lens, only capturing my outer appearance. I just had to fake it through a few more minutes and convince everyone that nothing was off. As the fire department's wellness coordinator, it was only logical that I be the one to give the interview for a story on post-traumatic stress in first responders. I explained to the reporter that post-traumatic stress was prevalent in first responders due to the nature of our jobs. Nearly every shift we worked, we saw traumatic events that the average person might see once or twice in a lifetime. In our profession, it was just another day. I labeled it *Tuesday*.

The interview wrapped up, and the camera was turned off. The lights dimmed and the reporter walked away with the microphone, yet I was still acting. The devastating truth was that while urging others to seek help if they were struggling, I was hiding that I had been silently suffering for a long time. I'd thought that maybe if I ignored it long enough, the pain would subside. But as time went on, the pain only grew, and I found myself at a dangerous new low. I had lost my way as well as my purpose. I was perpetually stuck in Tuesday.

It wasn't just the trauma from the fire world that had brought me to my knees. It was a culmination of that as well as childhood trauma, organizational betrayal, cancer, survivors' guilt, a superhero complex, moral injury, and mental health issues. I foolishly tried to carry the burden of all of these things, and it broke me.

When I was a child, my dad was gone a lot of the time due to his work schedule. I secretly craved his approval but went about gaining it in all of the wrong ways. I was rebellious and angry as a teenager, and my mom didn't know how to handle my defiance. The perfect storm of my misperception and anger resulted in a physical altercation with my dad, which left emotional scars that took decades to fade. I developed an insecurity that people would abandon me, and so I built walls around my heart, not only keeping others out, but keeping myself isolated from genuine relationships.

I loved my profession, but there were many things that I saw within it that I don't believe humans are meant to see, let alone witness over and over again. The violence, death, and evil I was exposed to took a toll on me, a little at a time. Once upon a time I stood as a young man, proudly donning dirty gear covered in soot. Now I stood as a middle-aged firefighter, the novelty worn off, the black ash painfully tarnishing my insides.

I poured my time and energy into making positive changes in the fire service regarding occupational cancer. At first, it felt as though I was finally where I was supposed to be. I was passionate, knowledgeable, and thrived while helping others create a healthier work environment. Then new leadership with a different agenda joined the organization. Without their support, I quickly went from being the one making a difference to the one trying to improve things in vain, and I was let go from the organization. I also held a leadership position where I assisted members struggling with mental health issues. Even though I tried to follow protocol to the best of my abilities, I was falsely accused of breaking confidentiality. Desperately in need of additional support, I received the cold shoulder instead.

Out of the blue, I was diagnosed with thyroid cancer. Thankfully we caught the cancer in a very early stage, and my doctors were able to remove it before it was too late. I struggled with the fact that I survived this deadly disease, yet some of my close friends had not been as lucky. I didn't understand why *I* was still standing and *they* were not. Why was my life spared, when they still had so many years ahead of them, so many more moments and days to live? I had a nagging fear that although I escaped death this time, it was only a matter of time before the cancer found its way back into my body.

Like many first responders, I took on a superhero persona, trying to save everyone around me. There were several problems with this, one being that there's not one person on the planet capable of saving all of the hurting people around them. This is why we must learn to rely on the strength of God. I had tunnel vision, only focusing on helping those around me who were struggling. I failed to acknowledge the way that I was slowly falling apart. It felt good being able to help others, but ultimately it ended up playing a huge role in the decline of my mental and physical health.

The combination of all of these things led me to a riveting mental health battle, one which almost cost me my life. I was plagued with deep depression, lost in seemingly endless darkness. In addition to that, I suffered from anxiety, certain that something horrific would happen each time I left the safety of my home. I still suffer from post-traumatic stress, as I don't think it truly ever goes away. It causes me to experience hypervigilance, insomnia and irrational concerns. There's a constant battle with the voices in my head that are urging me to give up and magnifying my fears. Relationships with those closest to me have slipped away, as I was too tired from acting as though I was fine to invest in people who deserved much more. I deserved much more too.

I had accrued an invisible set of armor that I thought would protect me and hide my vulnerable state from everyone. The armor was incredibly heavy, yet I took it everywhere, too ashamed to allow anyone to see how dire my situation had become. Despite my will for the invisible iron to stay intact, tiny cracks started to appear until the entire façade imploded. The act was up, and I was left exposed and broken in front of the ones I loved and lied to the most.

Not only had I overcome a battle with cancer and regularly dealt with dangerous on-the-job situations that could have claimed my life, I also experienced an attack on my character and lost people I loved. In spite of all this, I found a way back to my feet, until now. In an ironic twist of fate, I needed to be saved from *myself.*

The fight for my life has been the hardest battle in which I have ever engaged. At times, I honestly didn't know if I would make it out alive. God willing, I'm still standing. Though I have brokenness throughout me, I dare say I am stronger now because of it. God took these broken pieces and wove them together, and He uses my weaknesses to display His strength. I could easily tuck these struggles away and never look back, but I believe that my story has the potential to help others who are walking a trajectory similar to my past. I want to shed light onto the dark places that no one wants to acknowledge, because despite our reluctance to admit it, they exist.

I created a beautiful illusion of what I thought strength and resiliency looked like. It was never meant to withstand the true storms we experience in life. After the first big wave hit me, my world crumbled like a sandcastle caught in the tide. Everything I thought I knew was washed out from under me. It took a combination of therapy, medication, unwavering support from loved ones, and surrendering it all to Jesus for me to be able to start over and build a new, stronger foundation, meant to withstand the turbulence we experience in life. I know the hopeless feeling of your dreams and purpose being washed away into an endless abyss. While the waves will always be a part of the ocean, there is plenty of sand to use to rebuild, and the sun will always come out again. It can't stay dark forever.

My sister and I collaborated on writing this book. At first, I balked at the idea, knowing that my vulnerability would open me up for scrutiny and harsh judgement. Ultimately, the mission outweighed my insecurities, and we moved forward writing my story. If you know either of us, you will likely recognize that this is *my* story, in *her* words. She omitted my swear words, but the message of each chapter remains the same. The heartbeat behind this book is the desire that others will learn from the costly mistakes I've made in my personal life as well as my career and avoid repeating them in their own lives.

Along my journey, a few of the stories I am going to share might be disturbing to some. If certain content seems triggering, you may want to skip over that particular chapter, as this book is meant to help and not hinder you.

We wrote the stories in chronological order, so if it seems as though some of them don't flow together, it's because they don't. Parts of my life have been very messy and far from linear. The goal isn't to give you whiplash from the tumultuous highs and lows, but to give you an accurate depiction of the way events took place.

Not too long ago, I remember wondering if anyone would even miss me if I was gone. It seemed like it would have just been easier for everyone else if I was out of the equation. My pain had become a burden, not just to me, but to my family as well. I genuinely felt as though my story no longer mattered. I was wrong. My story does matter. Yours does too!

I promise you that hope *is* waiting on the other side, you just need to have the courage to ask for the help you've earned. Together we'll get through all of this pain, and tomorrow it won't be Tuesday.

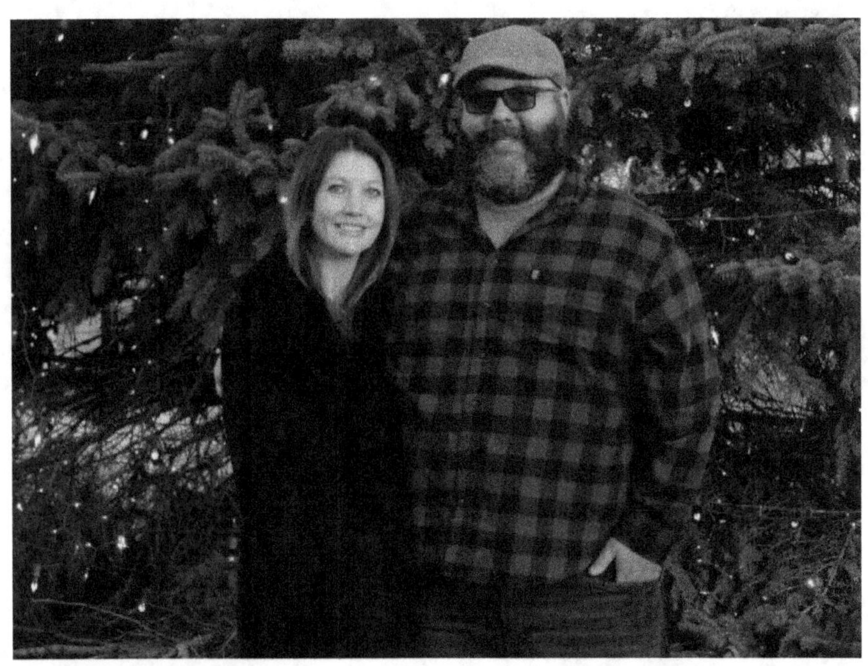

Hilary Hawkins & Jim Burneka Christmas 2023

2 – GROWING UP

Family dynamics can be tricky, and I think the majority of families who are honest would agree. I am the oldest of three siblings, with sisters three and six years younger than me. The good news is that the tumultuous relationships I experienced growing up have since been reconciled. The bad news is that it took quite a bit of time and therapy to get there.

My mom was a schoolteacher who taught special education for over thirty years. Although her job required immense energy and dedication, she always managed to get dinner on the table and arrange for three kids to get to three different sports practices (often at the same time.) She had summers off with us, so we always had a good time going to the pool and hanging out with our friends. We did the summer reading program and won Pizza Hut personal pan pizzas. We rode our bikes until dusk. We played in the treehouse my dad built. It was a really nice change of pace from the rest of the year.

My dad spent the bulk of his career in car sales, which is a tough business. A hard month means a small paycheck, regardless of the hours he spent pounding pavement on the lot. Whereas my mom stayed at the same school the majority of her teaching career, my dad moved car dealerships often. So often that he kept a cardboard box in the back of his trunk in case he decided it was time to leave his job on any given day. He worked long hours, and typically didn't come straight home from work. He liked to stop at the Red Carpet Tavern and have a beer to help him unwind before coming home. This resulted in him missing out on some of the household's day-to-day occurrences. We were going to bed by the time he walked in the door. When we were younger, he coached our t-ball/baseball teams, but as his job changed, his time constraints did as well. I will say that he always made an effort to show up at our games and special events.

I have had a quick temper ever since I was a little kid. It never took much to set me off, and once the fuse was lit, I exploded. It didn't really matter what caused it, and often the person who pulled the last straw was the recipient of my rage. I was pretty mean to my little sisters for no reason. They weren't exactly my biggest fans and usually just tried to stay out of my way. My dad was gone a lot of the time, so unfortunately, my mom was left dealing with my bad attitude and temper. My mom and I argued a lot, and there were several times she wanted to kick me out of the house. My dad would always tell her that throwing me out wasn't an option, and he would try to calmly talk to both of us. I slowly felt resentment building inside me toward my dad for being gone so often. It was true that he didn't have a steady salary and had to put in a lot of hours if he wanted to make money; what bothered me was that we weren't his first stop after leaving work. My mom would attempt to discipline me, but I never really took her seriously. When my dad would actually enforce whatever punishment my mom tried to delve out, I didn't respect what he was doing. Although I deserved it, I didn't always respond well to being disciplined.

There were a few physical altercations between the two of us. There was one explosive fight in particular that shifted the trajectory of my life. My mom and I were arguing about something and I was acting out of control. My mom yelled for my dad, who was in another room, to come in and help her. When my dad walked in, he was extremely angry with the way I was acting. My dad shoved me away from my mom, and we pushed each other a few times. We took a few swings at each other, and my dad clocked me right in the eye when I wasn't looking at him. Dad was typically the calm voice of reason, so it shocked me that he hit me so hard. My eye was painfully bruised and swollen. I could not believe our fight had escalated that far; fights between us never had before. We stopped speaking to each other and didn't talk for the next five-or six months, until my high school graduation. I had been working part-time and saving my money so that I could move out. That fight finalized my decision that I needed to get out of there. The day I graduated high school, I moved out of my childhood home into a house a few blocks away with three of my friends. We were all really young and threw a bunch of parties, relishing in our new-found freedom. At the time, one of the other guys in the house and I were attending college, and we realized that while our house was a lot of fun, it was not conducive to studying. After living there for about a year, we moved out and rented my grandma's house. I ended up buying that house and lived there for about 13 years.

A lot has happened since moving out of my parents' house. I will go more into detail in later chapters, but I ended up going through a lot of therapy and was encouraged to talk to my dad about some of the feelings I had stemming back from childhood. We had tough but good conversations that allowed us to move forward and enjoy our reconciled relationship.

My parents currently play a huge role in my life, as they are extremely active in my sons' lives as grandparents. Whereas my dad missed out on a lot of my activities as a kid, he shows up for everything my kids have. Soccer game in the rain? He's there. Basketball game an hour away? He's there. Baseball game on a sweltering hot day? He's there. Now that he's retired, he has a flexibility that didn't exist when I was a kid. His greatest joy is being with his grandkids, and it shows. I'm really glad that we were able to have some hard conversations that have allowed us to move on from the past and forge a new, stronger relationship. Not everyone gets this chance, so I would encourage you to talk to the people you love. It is never too late to mend fractured relationships!

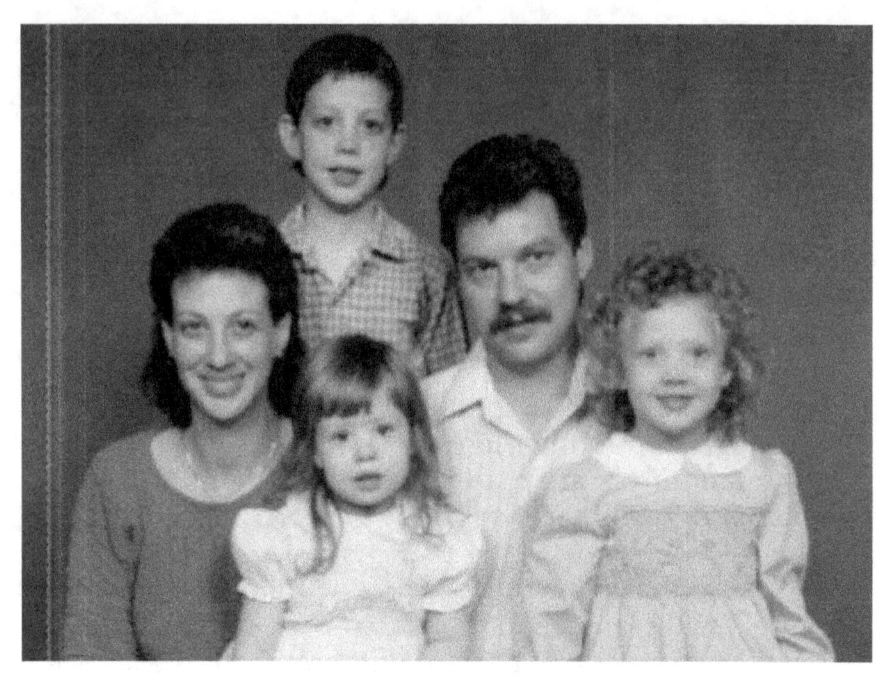

The Burneka's late 80's

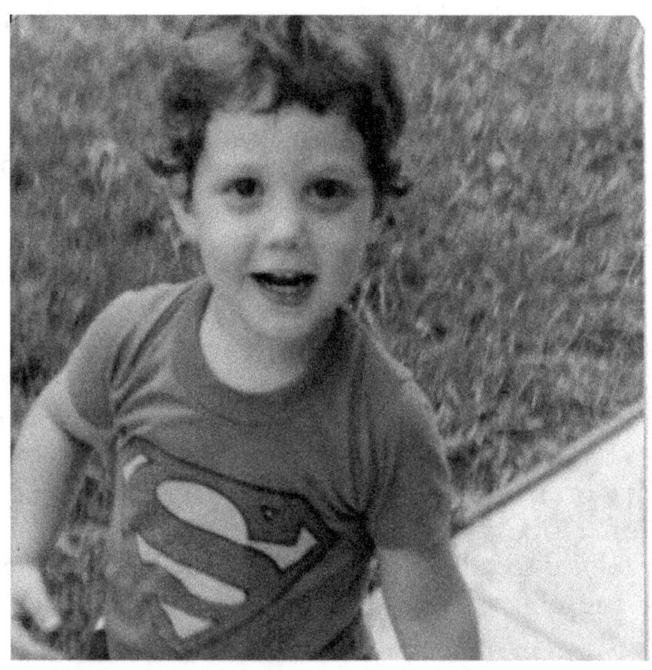

Back when I was cute

3 – INTRO TO THE FIRE SERVICE

"You don't have to see the whole staircase, just take the first step."
-Martin Luther King Jr.

When I was around fifteen or sixteen years old, it's safe to say I wasn't a model teenager. My grades were terrible, and I had a bad attitude and a hot temper to go along with it. I didn't know what my future held, but I knew a desk job or going to a fancy college weren't in the cards for me. I had just gotten a car, so if I wanted gas money, I needed to get a job.

My first job was working part-time at Hara Arena, a local arena where concerts, hockey games, wrestling competitions, and other events were held. I was hired on as an usher, so I basically got to watch all of these events for free. It was the perfect first job for me. During the summer I worked at a drive-in movie theater. I also worked at a few fitness stores. Those jobs served their purpose, but I was trying to figure out what piqued my interest, and what I was good at. I liked the jobs I had alright, but they weren't anything I found myself getting excited about. I didn't see a future in any of them.

Around the time I started driving, I got the opportunity to do a ride-along on a fire engine with one of my dad's friends, Jeff, who was a lieutenant. He took me to Station 13's, which was pretty busy. I went on a few calls with them, nothing crazy or significant, and then went back and hung out with the crew at the firehouse. It was like one big, extended family. I took in the comradery among the guys, and how they seemed to be having a good time at work, messing with each other and hanging out. They got the ladder truck out and let me climb the aerial ladder. I couldn't believe these guys found a profession where they *got paid* to hang out with their friends and go on adventures. No two calls were ever the same. This seemed like a dream job. All it took was the one visit and I was hooked. I didn't question my future anymore; I *knew* without a doubt that I was going to become a firefighter.

After I graduated high school, I took a first-level firefighter course at Sinclair Community College. After completing the class, I worked part-time at two different firehouses- one in Washington Township, and one in Harrison Township. The two could not have been more different. Washington Township was referred to as "the land of milk and honey." The stations were top-notch, with shiny new equipment and a firehouse equipped with all of the best furnishings. The community we served was quiet and relatively calm. Harrison Township was the polar-opposite. The station was run down, and they operated with older equipment. They didn't have the funds to maintain their station. The community was *not* quiet or calm. We stayed busy and responded to people in the lower socioeconomic status bracket. Harrison Township was the reality check that I needed after working at Washington Township. I credit my time at Harrison Township for preparing me for the City of Dayton Fire Department.

I wanted to get hired on in the City of Dayton, and fellow firefighters discouraged me from applying there. I continued to prepare to take their test, regardless of what everyone was telling me. The city publically discussed their goal of diversify the fire department. They wanted the first responders to reflect the community that they served. As a white male, I wasn't the demographic they were pursuing. Nevertheless, I applied for the job and took the City of Dayton fire test. I scored well on the test, and against all odds, I was hired.

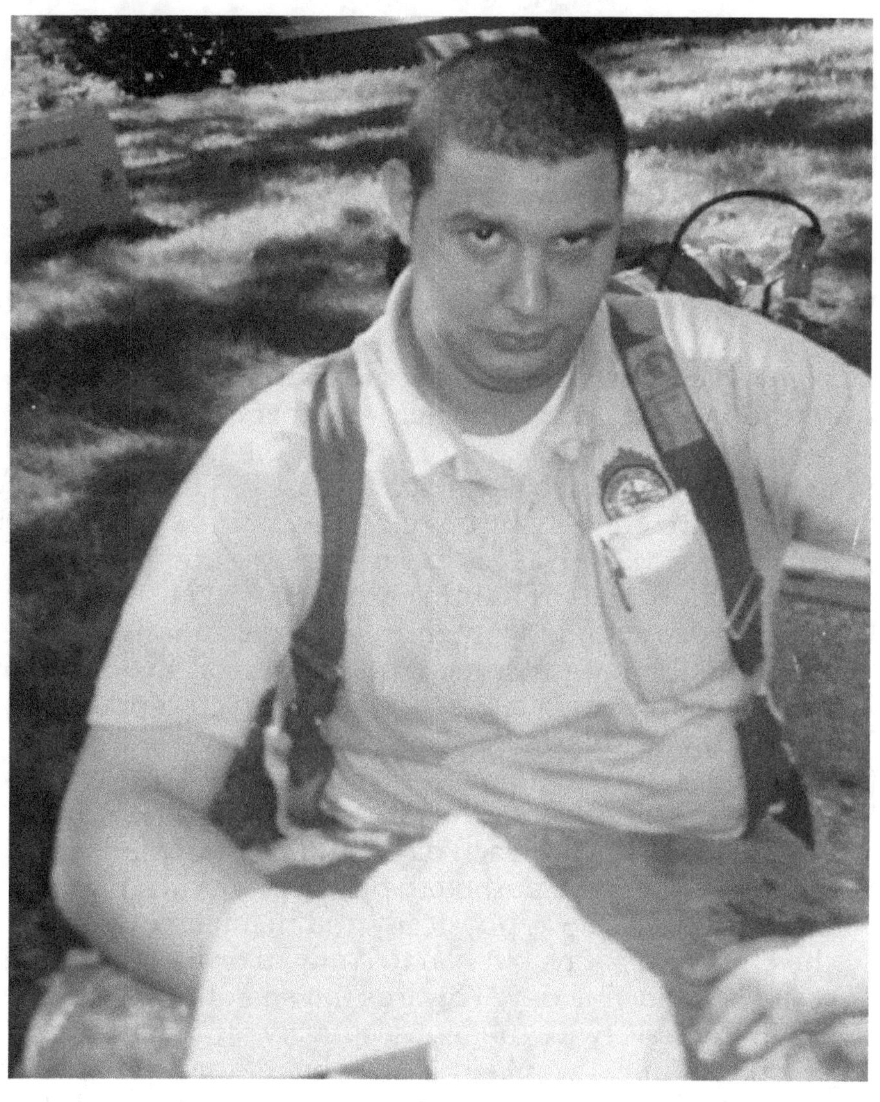

After my first structure fire sometime in 2000

4 – THE ACADEMY

"Do or do not. There is no try."
-Yoda

I had achieved my longtime goal of getting hired on with the City of Dayton Fire Department. Before I could begin working there, I had to go through the City of Dayton Fire Academy. They were short staffed, and the employees were working crazy overtime hours. In an effort to get some relief for their members, for the first time, they had two classes of twenty going through the academy simultaneously. I was in class B. The academy classes were Monday through Friday, starting January 29th and ending May 31st. This experience was nothing like the relaxed level-one firefighting class I had taken at Sinclair. It was overwhelmingly intense. The expectations were high, and there wasn't much room for error. Every day we had to take a written test, as well as complete a practical test (throw a ladder, tie a knot, operate a radio, etc.) If we failed our tests two weeks in a row or three weeks total, we would get kicked out of the program. It was a rigorous schedule, starting off each day with physical training, where we would be pushed to our limits in running and other exercises. I was physically and mentally exhausted at the end of each day, but had to study in order to pass the tests the following day. Towards the end of the academy, I failed my tests twice (not consecutively). If I failed a test one more time, I would be kicked out of the academy. The amount of stress and pressure I felt was staggering. If that wasn't enough, my girlfriend at the time broke up with me because I wasn't giving her enough attention. Of course, I know now that I was meant to be with my wife, but back then it really stung. The academy took every ounce of focus and energy I could muster. I was physically, mentally, and emotionally drained.

I quickly became very close to the other people in my class. We all worked together after we finished with the academy for the day, studying and preparing for the next day. We also encouraged each other through the physical training. I know that I wouldn't have gotten through the academy without their support. It is a unique experience to go through with other people, and due to the circumstances, we developed a close bond. I am still close today with a lot of the guys who were in the academy with me, and I'll always treasure the friendships that we formed there.

I was one bad week away from failing out of the academy, but with the help of my classmates and a lot of hard work, I made it through. When it was time to graduate, I was relieved and excited. My parents were in attendance, and I knew it was a really proud day for them. You have to remember; I'd been a pain-in-the-neck teenager who hadn't shown a lot of promise. But I had risen to the occasion and succeeded. I was finally going to get to do what I had wanted to do since I was a teenager, and I was ready to prove myself to the rest of the crew at the station. Maybe it was incredibly naïve, but I was filled with a hope and hunger to impact my community. At only twenty-one years old, I was ready to take on whatever would be thrown my way.

I was assigned to Station 15's, which ended up being both a blessing and a curse. It was great because the station was only three blocks from my house, and two blocks from where I grew up. I could easily navigate the streets during runs, even if I was half asleep. The downside, which I hadn't anticipated, was that I knew a lot of the people that we responded to on calls. If someone has to call 911, it's never for anything positive. I would go on to see people I had grown up with seriously injured or dead. I watched some grandparents of childhood friends die right before my eyes. It is hard enough to watch a person die, but when it's someone you have known since childhood, it takes a whole different toll on you. I remained optimistic, not realizing the effects from experiencing traumas didn't simply vanish into thin air. They would sneakily build inside of me. I would eventually come to learn that trauma must be processed in a heathy way, but that knowledge would come with age and experience. The academy trained me to protect and serve my community, but no course could prepare me for the horrors I would encounter.

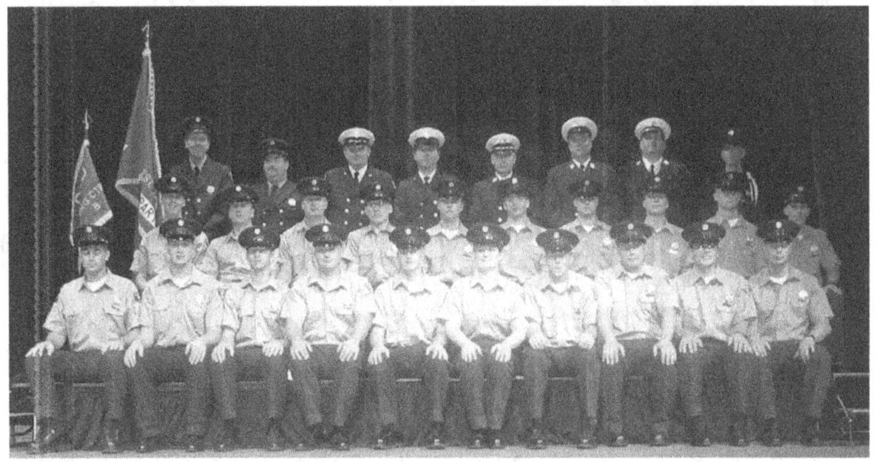

Dayton Fire Recruit Class 2001-B. I'm third from the right in the front row

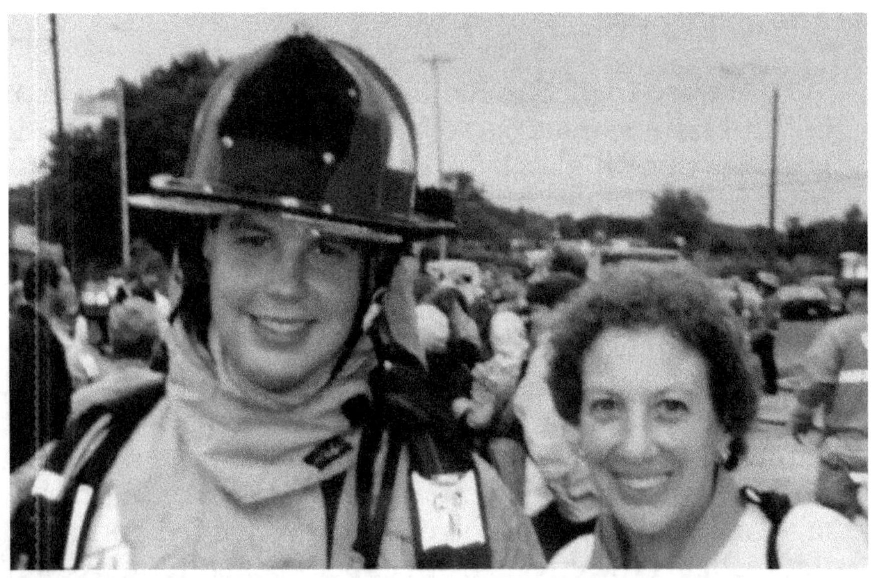

My mother and I on recruit academy graduation day

5 – FIRST DOSE OF REALITY

"There's no way around grief and loss: you can dodge all you want, but sooner or later you just have to go into it, through it, and hopefully come out the other side. The world you find there will never be the same as you left."
-Johnny Cash

I had just finished my probationary period and was finally allowed to take overtime shifts. At the time I wasn't married and didn't have any kids, so I was excited to make some extra money. I took an overtime shift at Station 16's riding the back of the engine. I was riding with a guy named Joe who'd graduated from the academy with me, so we were both relatively new to the job.

We were dispatched to a fire where people were trapped in the house. Joe and I were on the hose line. He was on the nozzle, and I was behind him. We were getting ready to go into the house when we saw a woman standing outside of the house. She hysterically told us that her baby was upstairs on the bed. She begged us to save her baby. I like pets as much as the next guy, but I was really hoping the baby she was referring to was an animal, not a human.

We were quickly able to locate the stairs and Joe swiftly put the fire out. I'm not sure what happened to our Lieutenant; he was supposed to be behind us but wasn't. Essentially, two rookies put out the fire.

In the same room the fire had been blazing, we found the baby. It was not a pet as I'd been hoping, but an actual human infant. Without going into too much detail, the baby was not alive and had been charred beyond recognition. It was easily the most horrific thing my eyes have ever seen. I can still picture it as though it was yesterday.

Since I was working overtime, I wasn't with my typical crew or station. Although the call bothered me to my

core, I couldn't show that finding the baby in that grue-
some condition had affected me. Basically, I couldn't show
any sign of humanity. We simply had to suck it up and
move on to completing overhaul. We never spoke about it
afterwards. This was the first of many similar calls that I'd
go on, just stuffing the trauma down, never showing any
emotion. We went back to the station and caught more
runs, pretty much pretending that it had never happened.
Let that sink in. I'd just witnessed the most horrific thing
in my lifetime and couldn't talk about it.

I will say, had this run happened today, the outcome
would've been different. Peer support would've been involved, and we would've had the option to talk about what
we'd experienced, or been allowed to leave our shift and
go home. It simply was not the culture back then.

This was a jolting wakeup call, that while the job
could be fun, I was going to see some messed up things
that no one should ever see. I had no way of understanding the vast realm of injuries and horrific situations I
would face. For the first time, I saw how dark the job—and
life—could be.

6 – THE JOB

This book touches on a lot of the heavy and dark aspects of my job. However, not everything I experienced in my job was traumatic. There were actually some pretty hilarious calls I went on and shenanigans that you just can't make up. I'm going to share some that are just so ridiculous you have to laugh.

The Help

When I was working at Station 11's, if there weren't enough people, they would take the engine out of service. I would either get stuck on the medic, or be sent to another station to ride on the engine there. It was a big hassle packing up all of my things and going to another station, so I was always a little annoyed when this happened. One day the engine at 11's was actually in service, and I was still sent to Station 16's. I was so mad that one of the few days the engine was in service, I had to leave. Nevertheless, I packed up all of my gear and headed over to Station 16's. While driving, I pulled onto the highway ramp too fast, and my car started going sideways. I'm not sure how, but I ended up flipping my car over on its side. Luckily, I had my seatbelt on, so I wasn't injured. I was able to release the seatbelt, and I was essentially standing up inside of my car. I got the window to roll down, and I pulled myself out of the car through the driver's side window. Mind you, I was wearing my Dayton Fire uniform. People who witnessed me flipping my car ran over in a panic. They asked if I needed them to call 911 and get help. I responded with, "I am 911." I told them I was fine, and there was no need to call 911. The last thing I needed was for my coworkers to see the mess I had just gotten myself into. But someone had to be the hero and call 911, and I saw my crew that I just left racing up the ramp. To make matters worse, they initially thought that I had witnessed the car flipping and pulled over to help. Once they realized it was *my* car that *I* flipped, they doubled over with laughter, taking pictures and roasting me. I ended up having the last laugh, though; since my car was wrecked, I ended up going back to Station 11's for the remainder of my shift, and someone else got shipped off to 16's.

The Draft

Ironically, this story took place right across the highway ramp from where I'd flipped my car. My partner, Pete, and I responded to a call where a driver had run his car into the highway wall. He didn't seem injured, but there was something off about him. The man was acting really squirrely. We were waiting for the police unit to arrive when he suddenly started to climb out of the window *Dukes of Hazard* style. He exited the car and was getting ready to jump over the wall, where there was a good thirty-foot drop. Pete and I jumped into action and grabbed him, throwing him on top of the car. We were on the radio calling for help, and the dude wouldn't stop fighting us. He was definitely under the influence of drugs, and it gave him superhuman strength. He bit Pete, and I wrestled with him on top of the car. It felt as if we were in a UFC fight on the side of the highway, right next to the wall where there was a thirty-foot drop. I stepped through the windshield while wrestling with this guy, and I finally was able to get him in an arm bar on top of the car. Once the police arrived, they pulled him off of the car and cuffed him. My partner and I still had to bring him to the hospital, and as I was walking down the hallway, I felt a really cool breeze on my butt. I was confused as to why I felt this random draft, and then realized that while we were wrestling on the car, the broken glass from the windshield had ripped my pants and underwear. I was casually walking around the emergency room with my bare butt exposed. I was so embarrassed! I was also mad, because my pants were new, and now I needed to pay to replace them. To top it off, because the guy bit Pete, we had to go to court and testify about the incident. It was really embarrassing at the time, but looking back on it, it's pretty hilarious (except the part where Pete got bit and being close to falling off the overpass).

Ebola

One summer evening we got a call regarding an ill man. We entered the house of the patient, and he was under a mound of covers, despite it being summer and not having air conditioning in the house. The man did not speak English. As my partner and I got closer to him, we saw that he was covered in bumps. My partner and I slowly backed out of the room, coming to the same horrible conclusion- there had recently been a rise in cases of Ebola virus, and we had just walked into a room with a man who was infected with it.

We called the hazmat team and waited for them to arrive and suit up before they could come in contact with the patient. We stayed in the medic and watched as they brought him out, tightly wrapped in a plastic-like wrap, looking like a human burrito. They loaded him into the medic, and we told the hospital that we were coming. They were ready for us when we arrived, and put all three of us together in an isolation room. My partner and I were furious that they put all three of us in isolation together. Finally, they put my partner and I in a room separate from the man. We were stuck waiting in the hospital all night. We Googled Ebola and learned all about the illness. By the end of the night, we were both convinced our deaths were imminent.

The hospital called in a specialist to test and examine the patient. Shortly after the specialist arrived, my partner and I were let out of our isolation room. We were released, free to go. It turns out that the man did not, in fact, have Ebola. He simply suffered from severe acne (hence the bumps all over his body) and was sick.

There are two serious things to take away from this story. The first one is that if you are in the fire service, or a first responder, be sure to communicate with your significant other about the calls you are experiencing at work. My wife had no idea that I had spent the night awake in isolation at the hospital. She and I started bickering about something silly, and when I told her what I'd just been through, she was understanding and gave me some space. The other thing is that whether it is Ebola or some other scary virus, do yourself a favor and do not research it on the internet! We were definitely looking at worst-case scenarios, and although we were cleared from the possibility of contracting Ebola, we heightened the stress of the situation by reading into something that didn't even exist. Be careful what you fill your mind with!

Medic Mayhem

My partner, Mike, and I were in the same class, but he became a medic before I did. I was working on becoming a certified paramedic, and I had to complete a certain number of runs being the lead paramedic. Since Mike was already checked off as a medic, he just had to basically babysit me and check off what I was doing. We were on the medic one day, and Mike was having an off day. He was taking out-of-the-way routes to calls. He seemed kind of all over the place, which isn't how he typically is. By the end of the day, I was super annoyed with him. We had a run that was by the University of Dayton, so we headed that direction. The engine was already at the house we were going to, making our destination very obvious. However, Mike drove right past where we were supposed to go. He turned around and drove back to the house, and I was fed up. I started talking trash to him, asking him what his problem was and why he drove past the house when there was already an engine there. I was half kidding, but also half serious.

He had enough of my mouth, and I know that because he punched me in the face. I reacted and elbowed him, catching him in the mouth. He punched me again, and I headbutted him. If you haven't ever been in the front of the medic, there isn't a lot of room. We couldn't have an all-out brawl, so we resorted to punching, elbowing and headbutting each other (like five-year-olds). We stopped and stared at each other, both of us still really mad, but also realizing we needed to go inside of the house for the run we'd been dispatched to. We both exited the medic and stomped up to the house, both of us completely disheveled, with messed-up hair and wrinkled clothes. Mike's lip was bleeding. I'm sure we were both breathing heavily. The guys on the engine could tell something had gone down between us, but they knew better than to ask. We did our job and then left the scene. We talked out our frustrations and moved on. There wasn't a long and drawn-out hostility between us. If anything, we grew closer because we gained respect for each other. Mike and I are still good friends; I actually just played poker at his house a few days ago.

This happened twenty years ago, and I know that this kind of behavior would never fly these days. Someone definitely would've reported us, and we would've gotten in a lot of trouble. I'm not proud of this behavior or condoning violence, but it was just so ridiculous that it makes me laugh looking back on it. I kind of wish I could've seen what we looked like walking up to the call after hitting each other moments before. Just another night on the medic in Dayton.

Rumors and Showers

I had torn my ACL two times—my left knee playing basketball, and my right knee kicking in a door at a fire. The third ACL tear made me infamous around the firehouse—third time's a charm, right? It was New Year's Day and I decided that I would get to the station early to shave, shower, and get ready. The station in question is an older station. I was in the shower and the next thing I knew, the water turned scalding hot. It felt like lava was pouring down on me. I tried to jump out of the water stream as fast as I could, and in doing so I slipped and fell. As soon as I fell, I knew I'd torn my ACL again. I stayed on the shower floor for a minute, knowing that I was doomed.

Eventually, I was able to get up, hobble out of the shower, and get myself dried and dressed. I limped into the office that was next to the bathroom and called Boomer to come and help me. After I called him, I realized that he had flushed the toilet, and that was the cause in the sudden change in the water temperature. He helped me gather up my things and I called the district chief, explaining the situation and telling him I was heading to the hospital. He looked at the schedule and told me that I wasn't even on the schedule for the day. So, basically, I came in and tore my ACL on my day off. That was a pretty bitter pill to swallow.

Have you ever heard the saying "Never let the truth get in the way of a good story"? Well, rumors started circulating about what had happened to me, and my favorite one is that I burned my penis in the shower, and the medic crew had to take me to the hospital. I haven't confirmed or denied the rumor. I guess now everyone will know that all I did was slip and tear my ACL again.

Rollin'

Someone thought it would be funny to start a rumor that the one and only Limp Bizkit would be coming to Dayton and playing at a local Sunoco gas station. Although it was completely false, the graphics and social media posts looked pretty legitimate. A lot of people were convinced that the band was coming. It created such a buzz that Limp Bizkit actually had to release a statement saying they weren't coming to Dayton, and that it was just a rumor.

The evening that they were supposedly coming into town, a lot of people showed up at the gas station, despite

Limp Bizkit themselves shutting down the rumors. There were so many people there that the gas station had to close, and police officers were called to monitor the crowd.

I had picked up an overtime shift that night and was riding the medic with Boomer. We had just transported a patient to the hospital, and we were on our way back to the station. On our way back, we passed the Sunoco gas station, and while we were stopped at a red light, we decided to give them the concert they were all waiting for. We played Limp Bizkit's song "Rollin'" through the medic's PA speaker. Everyone thought it was hilarious and started waving their arms in the air. We might have been waving our arms in the medic too.

This could be one of those stories that you had to be there to truly understand how funny it was, but I still think that it's pretty good. It is most definitely not what the speakers on the medic were intended for, but a little fun never hurt anyone. We couldn't resist rocking out to some of their songs in light of the huge crowd that had gathered, waiting for a band that was never going to come.

I wanted to share some lighthearted stories, because there were a lot of joyous moments within the years that I worked. We laughed a lot, together and at each other. But just as there were highlights we loved to reflect upon, there were very dark moments as well. I'm going to share some of the heavier aspects I've experienced at work. It's time to throw the rose-colored glasses aside and see the dim reality we faced on the job.

7 – SNAKEBIT

"Snake's poison is life to the snake; it is in relation to man that it means death."
-Maulana Rumi

I had the day off and planned on tackling some work around the house. One of the guys that was on shift let me borrow his truck so I could haul materials from Home Depot. After I was done using his truck, I drove it back to the station. When I pulled up, everyone was standing outside by a parked van. Next to the van, there was a man lying on the ground. I didn't know what had happened, but I knew it wasn't good.

I was going through medic school, and as long as there was another medic present, I was allowed to help work on him. I was pretty new, so I didn't realize it, but the unconscious man was an active Dayton Firefighter. He had an extensive snake collection, and while he was feeding his snakes, he was bitten by one, a Rhinoceros Pit Viper. They are poisonous and look plain evil. They literally have horns on top of their heads (hence having *rhinoceros* in their name).

As soon as the snake bit him, he told his girlfriend, and they ran out the door to go to the hospital. He lived about five blocks from the station, and he had passed out by the time she drove the five blocks. When she pulled into the station, he was unresponsive and unconscious. The medic at 15's was out on a run, so we had to wait for the medic from 11's to come. I rode in the back with him to Miami Valley Hospital. The emergency room knew we were coming, and they were rapidly working to get him some antivenom.

The doctor at the hospital needed to identify the snake that bit him, so Tim Harrison, a firefighter and police officer who deals with wildlife in the area, went to his house and retrieved the snake. He brought it to the hospital in a plastic tote, and they brought the snake into the room with the man who had been bitten. The snake was going crazy inside of the tote, trying to escape. We could hear him banging his head against the lid, causing the tote to move. The thrashing intensified the longer the snake was trapped inside the tote. I didn't trust the plastic to hold up and didn't want to be anywhere near the snake.

Unfortunately, our fellow firefighter died from the snakebite. We had to go to a critical incident stress debriefing (CISD), and we were all beating ourselves up for not being able to save him. We did all that we could do, and it wasn't enough. It was a truly awful feeling. We were later told that the emergency room doctor determined that the snake bit right into a vein in-between the guy's thumb and pointer finger. It was essentially an IV push of venom, straight into his vein. Even if we'd been able to administer the antivenom as soon as it happened, it wouldn't have saved him. It was difficult to accept, but despite our best efforts, nothing would've changed the outcome. The defeat you feel after losing someone is monumental. I was learning the deep despair associated with death, and would soon learn the fear of my crew and I almost losing our own lives.

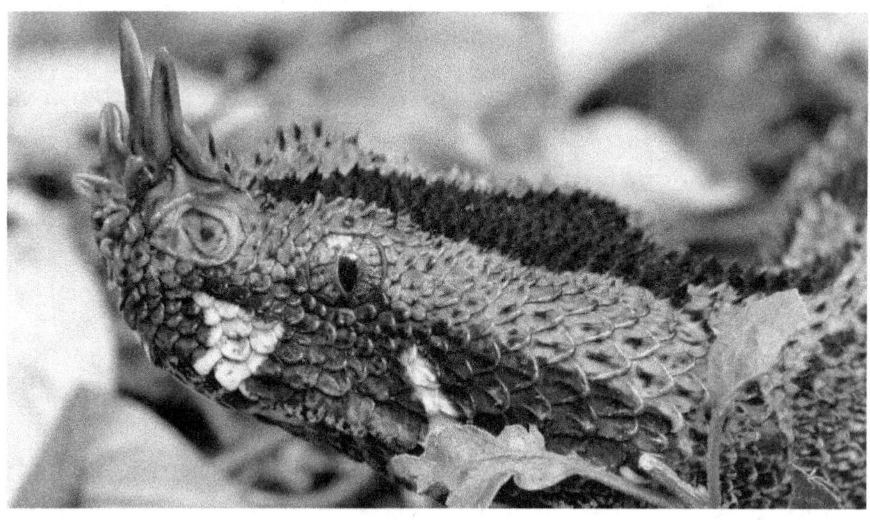

Rhino Pit Viper (photo courtesy of the Virginia Zoo)

8 – ISOTEC

I picked up an overtime shift on September 21st, 2003. I'd be working at the station that handles the bulk of hazmat calls in our district. We were dispatched to a call at the Isotec chemical manufacturing plant, where there was a nitric oxide leak. The building was located in Miami Township, which is about twelve miles south of Dayton. There were ten of us on the hazmat team, as well as guys from Miami Township on scene.

The hazmat coordinator briefed us on the situation and explained that if the building exploded, a poisonous cloud would form. If anyone breathed in the poisonous air, it would cause *automatic* asphyxiation. That was pretty alarming information to digest. I wasn't really nervous up until that point, but I think the new information was intimidating enough to unnerve anyone.

We spent the majority of the day at the Isotec plant while they tried to stop the leak. The Dayton chief and some other members went to do a lap outside of the Isotec facility. We were waiting for them to return. The next thing I knew, the building blew up. It happened in slow motion and fast, all at the same time. The explosion looked like it was from a movie. There was a bright flash of light, and a deafening blast that was low and deep. Windows blew out, and broken glass flew through the air and sprinkled across the ground like raindrops. Chunks of metal and concrete shards were propelled dangerously through the air. I ran faster than I'd ever run in my life to the hazmat truck and ducked behind it, covering my head with my arms. The people inside of the hazmat truck started coming out, donning self-contained breathing apparatuses (SCBAs) and protective gear so they could go look for our chief and the other members that had gone to do a lap outside of the building. I ran into the vehicle to grab a SCBA, but they were all gone. I knew if I breathed in any of the poison from the explosion, it would kill me. Without any face protection, I ran towards the medics, away from the billowing smoke slowly engulfing the sky.

Thankfully our chief and the other members were away from the building before it exploded. Although no firefighters were injured, it was easily the most intense call I had ever been on. In twenty-two years on the job, this was the most scared I've ever been. I know that with a lot of these calls, you really can't get a feel for how horrifying they are unless you experience them yourself. Trust me when I tell you that being in close proximity to an exploding building, with poisonous gas filling the air, is utterly terrifying. Not to mention, thinking our crew was severely injured or killed. Words cannot possibly express the fear I felt during all of this.

I entered the shift thinking it was Sunday and I was going to have a pretty relaxed day. I couldn't have been more wrong. No amount of overtime pay was worth the stress and danger we encountered on this run! I was grateful for my union role as the special events coordinator. The position allowed me to shift my focus from terror associated with work to planning uplifting events that could bring a moment of happiness to others within my fire family. It was time to shift my fear-focused thoughts into something positive.

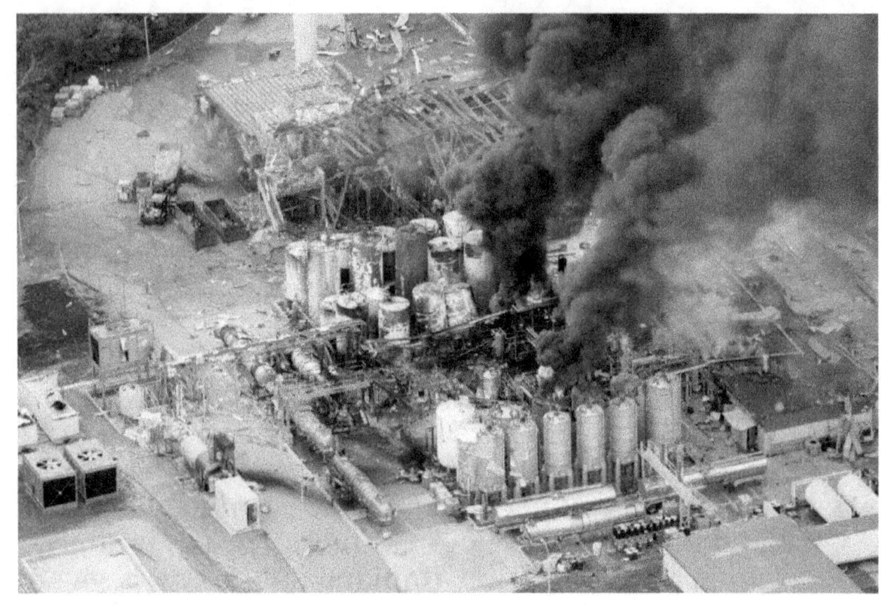

Aftermath of the Isotec explosion (photo courtesy of the
Dayton Daily News)

"The world ain't all sunshine and rainbows. It's a very mean and nasty place, and I don't care how tough you are; it will beat you to your knees and keep you there permanently if you let it. You, me, or nobody will be hit as hard as life, but it ain't about how hard you hit, it's about how hard you can get hit and keep moving forward."

-Rocky Balboa – Rocky Balboa

Sean Lucas is a fellow firefighter and close friend of mine. In 2006, his five-year-old son, Gavin, was diagnosed with Ewing's Sarcoma, a rare type of cancer that forms in the bones or soft tissue. I was devastated for Sean and vowed to do anything I could to help him through this difficult time.

I was serving as the union special events coordinator when Gavin got sick. I couldn't cure his cancer, so I did what I knew how to do well—I started planning events to support them. The first event I put together was a shave-in. We held this at a local bar called Flanagan's. At this point, Gavin had lost all of his hair, so a bunch of us were going to shave our heads in solidarity. A lot of firefighters participated in this event, showing their support for Sean and Gavin. I can't think of a lot of other professions where the brotherhood is so strong people would be lined up to voluntarily shave their heads for the sake of a five-year-old.

At the same venue, we put together a huge Guitar Hero concert/benefit. (I know I am aging myself with this story. Trust me, it used to be very cool!) All of the local news and radio stations were involved in covering and promoting this event. The bar was jam packed with a sea of people wearing navy blue Team Gavin t-shirts. Team Gavin rubber bracelets adorned many wrists in the crowd. We were fortunate enough that a lot of local businesses donated items and gift cards to raffle off. There were a lot of really cool prizes that were available to win. We had a dance-off, and a few friends and I actually performed a choreographed dance we rehearsed to an NSYNC song. We crushed it. My good friend Rod played the guitar and sang. There were so many people that jumped in and happily lent their talents to help us pull off the event. Rotating shifts of volunteers helped with everything from Guitar Hero gaming to selling raffle tickets. If you've ever seen an Irish bar on St. Patrick's Day, you'd know the crowd is huge. The crowd for our event was just as plentiful, if not more so. Pat Flanagan (the owner) said it was the most soda he's ever served in a single day. It was a bittersweet event. The reason we threw it was heartbreaking, but watching our fire family and local community show up in such a big way was pretty incredible.

Team Gavin included firefighters, family, and friends. But it was much bigger than that. Complete strangers were pulling for Gavin to beat the sickness that consumed his tiny body. We were flooded with support from people all over the country, standing in the gap for Sean's family, bolstering their spirits with hope. (I know some of you will be wondering, and I'm elated to tell you that Gavin has now been cancer-free going on eighteen years, and he's doing great!)

The benefit exceeded the monetary goals we'd set, and Sean declined accepting the extra money. He wanted it to go to organizations affiliated with cancer, so we researched various options. We ended up donating to two non-profits- Cure Search and the Firefighter Cancer Support Network (FCSN). We were familiar with Cure Search but discovered the FCSN by a random Google search.

I didn't realize it at the time, but our Google search led me to a significant role I'd soon be stepping into. Many times we don't understand why things happen, but the reasons are eventually revealed down the road.

Me, Hilary, Sean, Gavin & Valerie

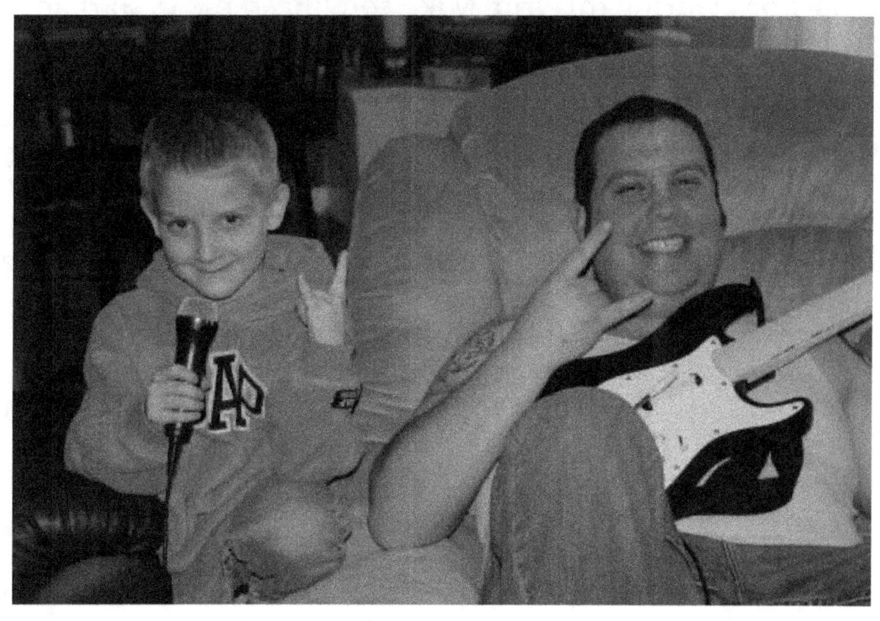

Gavin and I playing some rock band

10 – A PASSION IGNITED

"Passion is kind of important for me, whether it's playing sports or whether it's just living or whatever you're going to do. In my opinion you should be passionate about it or else, why do it?"
-Pat Tillman

On behalf of Team Gavin, we cut a check to the FCSN. They were a brand-new nonprofit organization based out of Southern California, so they were extremely appreciative and shocked to receive a random donation from a small town in Ohio. Mike Dubron, the president and founder of FCSN, flew to Dayton and attended one of our union meetings to show his sincere gratitude.

During my extra days off (EDOs), I started visiting every Major League ballpark in the U.S. My next stop was in California, and Mike offered to pick me up from the airport. During this trip, Mike convinced me to start and direct the first Ohio Chapter of the FCSN.

My role as director of the Ohio Chapter was to educate firefighters on how significant of a threat cancer is to us. At the time, this was a taboo subject that was awkward to talk about. The new information I was relaying to firefighters wasn't exactly received well. I quickly learned that most of us (myself included) felt as though we were pretty invincible. It's part of the mindset we tap into during our shifts. Let's face it, we are frequently confronted with extreme situations. We need to be confident and unafraid in the midst of these events. But the reality is that the same mentality that helps us complete our job hurts us when it comes to our own health and wellbeing.

I continued my quest to share knowledge and information regarding occupational cancer. On my thirtieth birthday, I was promoted to vice president of regions. This meant that I oversaw all the state coordinators. I did this for a few years until the president stepped down. The board elected me to fill the vacant spot as interim president. My goal was to simply ensure that what Mike had started not only stayed afloat but thrived in his absence.

I was in the role of president for about six months. During this time I expanded the board, submitted an Assistance to Firefighters Grant (AFG), and notably, we created the FCSN Whitepaper. The FCSN Whitepaper was a report that expanded upon how significant of a threat cancer is to firefighters, how to take action against cancer in the fire service, and practical steps to take to reduce the risks of getting cancer.

The FCSN found a new permanent president, and I resumed my role as the director of the Ohio Chapter. The grant proposal I'd submitted while I was in the president's role was awarded to the FCSN. I'd started to notice the board doing things that weren't included in the grant. I became very vocal about this, as *my* name was the one in the grant. Since I submitted it, I knew the specific amount of money that was allocated to different areas. I continued to speak up about the discrepancies, despite knowing I was going against the grain.

I was in charge of mailing out the supplies for the FCSN, and one day the corporate credit card I used was declined at the post office. I figured there was probably just an error with the bank and didn't think too much of it. Then a little later, I received a certified letter from the FCSN stating that my talents and services were no longer needed.

I was in disbelief that I'd been fired from a volunteer position. It was humiliating, to say the least. Aside from my embarrassment, I was angry. I'd thrown so much of my time and effort into this organization, and not only believed in the work they were doing, but I'd also become super passionate about their mission. I assumed that all of the positive contributions I'd made didn't outweigh the trouble I caused by calling out the misuse of the grant.

Looking back, I was still pretty immature. I had great intentions, but my actions didn't always reflect them. This was the first brush with organizational betrayal that I would experience through my career. If you are unfamiliar with the term, organizational betrayal is a deep violation of trust that occurs when an organization fails to protect an employee that is dependent upon their support.

My involvement with the FCSN ignited a passion within me I didn't even know I possessed. Ironically, caught up in my turmoil and anger, I started a fire and threw in every FCSN-related item I owned. I watched the shirts and items burn in the flames, until just like my hopes, they were reduced to mere ashes.

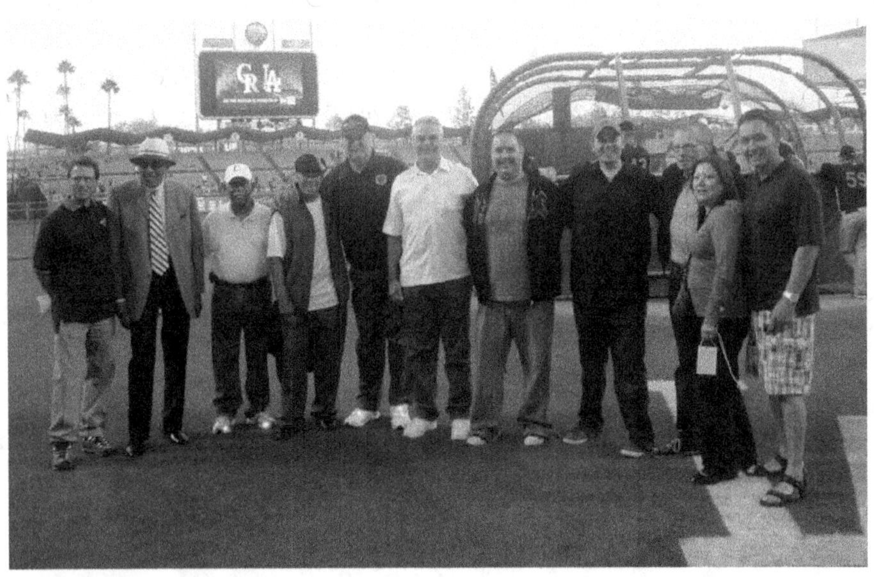

FCSN members with Larry King at Dodger Stadium

11 – LAUREN

"To be fully seen by somebody, then, and be loved anyhow—this is a human offering that can border on miraculous."
-Elizabeth Gilbert

In my professional life, things may have been a mess, but in my personal life, I had one person that was always a constant—my wife, Lauren. I've known her for almost as long as I can remember. Growing up, I was friends with her twin sisters, who are four years older than her, and we all went to the same grade school. Lauren was always around, but I didn't really pay much attention to her when we were kids because she was so much younger.

I stayed close with her family throughout high school, despite her sisters and I going to different high schools. Lauren and I developed a friendship, and I took Lauren to her high school prom. We remained friends, and around my thirtieth birthday we started dating. There was something different about Lauren that drew me in, and I really liked spending time with her. Being the romantic that I am, I asked her to be my girlfriend at an Alice Cooper concert. (I know what you're thinking, and I'm not sure why she said *yes* either.)

I was already working for the Dayton Fire Department, and Lauren was still in college. There was no doubt in my mind that she was the person I wanted to spend the rest of my life with. While I was visiting my grandma in Florida, she told me that she wanted to give me her wedding ring to use for Lauren's engagement ring. Creating a custom, vintage-looking ring complete with my grandma's diamond was the perfect sentimental gesture Lauren would appreciate. I began to plan my proposal, getting a little help from my sister and her husband. It had to be a memorable night for Lauren, so we went to visit my sister and brother-in-law where they lived in St. Louis. We arranged for a horse-drawn carriage to pick us up and take us to dinner. Lauren and I enjoyed the picturesque carriage ride through downtown St. Louis, taking in the unique buildings and liveliness of the city. The carriage driver wore a suit and a top hat, and it really felt as though we were in a movie. The carriage dropped us off at the Millennium Hotel, and we took an elevator all the way up to the top of the building, to the Top of the Riverfront restaurant. It was an upscale, spinning restaurant that overlooked all of downtown St. Louis, including the iconic arch. I asked a woman at the table next to us if she would take our picture, and then I dropped down on one knee and proposed to Lauren. I could not have been more ecstatic that she said yes.

We planned an outdoor wedding in August, and the day of our wedding the weather was perfect. All of our friends and family were there, and my good friend Rod officiated the ceremony. It wasn't a huge ceremony, but we did include our close friends and families. Lauren did a great job planning all the small details, expressing our personalities throughout the wedding. Speaking of personalities, I had a small lapse in judgement in planning our transportation from the wedding to the reception hall. I wanted to surprise Lauren, so I arranged to have a helicopter pick us up from the wedding venue and take us to the reception hall. I thought Lauren would love this big romantic gesture, but I didn't account for the wind and her wedding dress. Or her hair and makeup, which apparently took a lot of time and planning. Whereas I love to do things a little differently and sometimes over the top, Lauren doesn't share the same sentiment. Let's just say that during the helicopter ride Lauren was up in the air, but not exactly swept off her feet.

Lauren works as a pediatric nurse and is the most compassionate person I know. She's definitely who you'd want taking care of your child! She has an innate kindness that's unmatched. Lauren's the most incredible mother to our two boys, Jameson and Logan. She's largely unselfish and always puts herself last. Lauren goes out of her way for everyone, always helping without being asked. We've had our shares of up and downs, but she has loyally stuck by my side. I know that I haven't been an easy partner, to put it lightly. I've unintentionally put her through the wringer. She has upheld our wedding vows, time and time again, sticking by me through times of sickness and health. Throughout our marriage, I've sustained injuries that have required surgery, received a cancer diagnosis, and suffered from mental illness. Lauren supported me through it all, the physical ailments as well as mental sickness. For a period of time, I was not myself, and became moody, unpredictable, and overly emotional. Most people would have left, and truthfully, I wouldn't have blamed them. Without her support, I don't know where I'd be right now. I don't say it enough, so, Lauren, thank you for your unwavering devotion.

I'm grateful we started our marriage with such a firm foundation. Future events were certain to shake us, but we were able to withstand the blows by sticking together. Just as our honeymoon had quickly passed, the honeymoon at work was also about to come to an end.

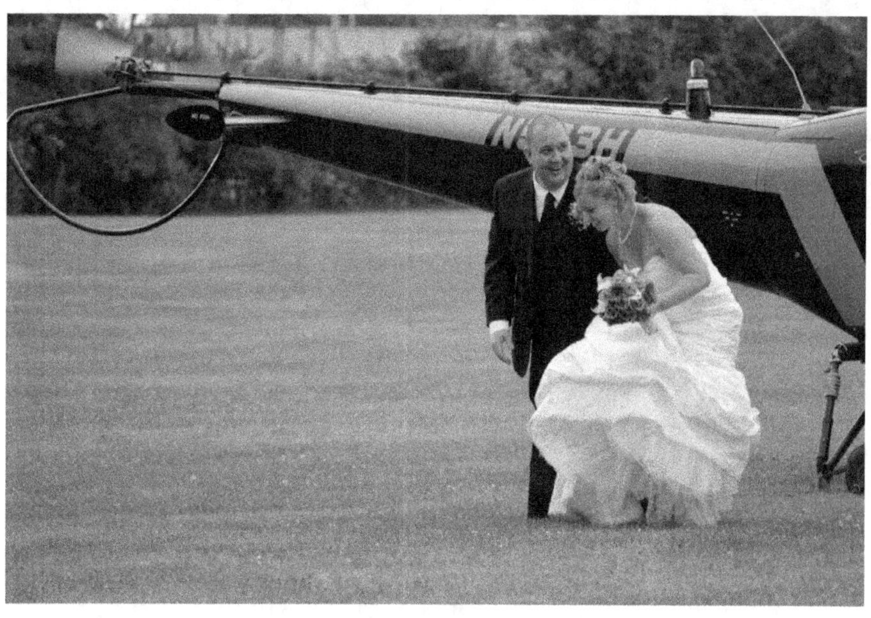

After the helicopter ride (notice her hair is fine)

"If I knew I was going to live this long, I'd have taken better care of myself."
- Mickey Mantle

I was transferred from Station 8's to 18's. I was happy at 8's, but I liked the crew over at 18's, so I was fine with moving there. The captain from 18's was training new recruits at the training center, so the relief captain (RC) filled in for him.

I know it varies across stations, but in Dayton, the protocol is to start off each shift with roll call at 0700 in the morning. This was when we would receive our assignments and duties for the shift and be given the rundown of the day.

My first day at 18's, the shift that worked before us was packing up their things to leave. RC addressed me in front of the crew getting ready to leave and my new crew and said, "I've been tasked with getting you in shape. How much do you weigh, anyway?" I answered honestly, and told him somewhere in the upper two hundreds. He proceeded to tell me that no one would be able to pull me out of a fire, and I was a hazard to myself as well as my crew. RC gave me orders to work out every day I was on shift. He threatened me that if I didn't work out, I'd be assigned to working on the medic. Working on the medic is an unofficial punishment in Dayton.

I was so embarrassed that he'd called me out in front of everyone. It was no secret I was overweight. This is a struggle I am well aware of. Thanks to my new captain, now everyone at Station 18's was aware of it too. Might I add, I'd been there all of one minute when all this took place. Welcome to Station 18's!

The harassment continued as RC privately pulled me into his office. He proceeded to ask me if I had a life insurance policy. I was confused why he was randomly asking me this, but answered that, yes, I have a policy through the city. He replied with, "Good, I'm sure that after you die one of these firefighters will enjoy burning through your money with your wife." I wanted to punch him in the mouth but bit my tongue and left the room. Most people would've struggled with trying to keep their cool in that moment. He could've made his point a thousand other ways, and I was disgusted by his approach.

I began working out on my shift days, but it was difficult to get a good workout in without being interrupted by calls. I thought I'd be able to work out more efficiently at home without interruption, so I started to wake up early and exercise before heading to work.

One day at work, RC asked me if I had exercised yet that day. I told him that I woke up early and rode my stationary bike at home before coming in for my shift. He asked if my wife saw me ride the bike, to which I replied yes. He asked for her phone number, and I thought he was messing with me. I gave it to him, and he actually called her. He left Lauren a voicemail that said something along the lines of, "Hey, this is RC, Jim's captain at 18's. I am just calling to confirm that Jim worked out this morning. Please call me back." I didn't know that he actually called Lauren until I received a text from her, confused over the whole interaction. I asked her if she called him back and if she kept the voicemail. She replied *yes* to both questions. I was livid. He'd crossed the line. Truthfully, none of what he was doing was okay. He was harassing me over my weight, and everyone knew it. But calling my wife? That was the last straw.

I called a meeting with my union representative, the district chief, RC, and the captain of 18's he was filling in for. I stated my case with documentation showing exactly what RC had said to me, when he said it, and the people that witnessed it. No one could argue with the facts I laid out. I had told my union rep that if I started to get too emotional or angry to pinch me. There were several times that my emotions began growing heightened, and he did actually pinch me to bring me back down. I noticed that the district chief was acting uncharacteristically aloof during our meeting. Then he became adamant that this issue become resolved right then and that I didn't escalate it any further. I thought his behavior was strange, until it clicked into place. RC had announced that "he was tasked" with getting me in shape. He directly reports to the district chief. I connected the dots that the district chief was the one who had ordered him to get on me about my weight. RC owned up to everything that I had stated happened and apologized. He assured me that the harassment would stop. The chief asked us if we were good. We both said we were good and agreed to move forward. I was relieved it was over, but frustrated it had taken place at all.

I want to make a few things clear. Part of firehouse culture is to roast each other and talk trash to each other. I have done my fair share of this. What I had been experiencing with RC wasn't funny or meant in a joking manner. It was a whole new level of bullying that I simply wouldn't endure once it involved my wife. That being said, he was right about me needing to lose weight. I *was* a risk to myself and my crew in a fire at my then-current weight. It wasn't his message that deeply cut me, but how he chose to say it. If he had pulled me aside and told me that he was concerned about my weight and wanted to help me come up with a workout and nutrition plan, I would've been receptive to it. I'd been struggling with my weight for quite some time. Having someone come alongside me and encourage me would've gone a long way. The way that he chose to approach the problem didn't motivate me to lose weight, but it did cause me to lose things. I lost my trust in my boss, as well as his boss. I lost respect from my crew due to his constant bullying in front of all of them. I lost confidence in myself to do my job well. I lost any bit of enjoyment in doing my job during that time.

Looking back, I know that RC is not a bad man. I believe that he truly had my best interests at heart. I don't think that his purpose was to humiliate me but to open my eyes to the grave reality that my weight was a danger to myself and others. If I didn't do something about it, I wouldn't be around to enjoy my wife and kids. I'd come to understand that a big part of my struggle with weight was how I was self-medicating with emotional eating.

When dealing with people and health issues, berating them won't disarm them and motivate them to change their habits. We've got to create a healthy culture where we come alongside each other when one of us is struggling, and we show up for them in a way that will benefit them. This taught me a valuable lesson moving forward in how to approach people in a respectful manner when addressing difficult issues. I don't always have a filter in what I say, so it did help me to be mindful about what I was saying. Our words carry more weight than we think. I'm proof that we just never really know what people are going through.

It's a good thing we were able to get all of that behind us, because the drug epidemic that was coming would consume the bulk of our mental capacity. We wouldn't have the energy to argue with one another; we were heading straight into the forefront of a drug war.

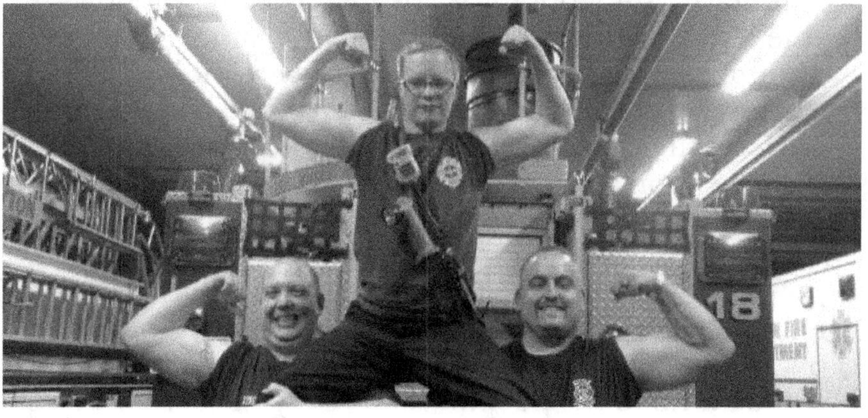

2nd Ammendment representing

13 – THE HEROIN DIARIES

"Stay away from drugs. They're not worth it. I've tried, but there's none of them that's worth it."
-Randy Newman

When I was working at Station 18's, we experienced a heroin epidemic. Between the years 2010 and 2015, Ohio became the drug overdose capital of the nation. Dayton (where I worked) was among the top ten cities in the nation for high drug overdose rates. The location of Ohio makes it an epicenter for drug distribution. Three main interstates run through Ohio: I-70, I-75 and I-80. Drug traffickers prefer the convenience and speed that are found on these major highways, making them a hotspot for drug dealers and their customers.

This epidemic put an enormous amount of stress on first responders. The station where I was working was in the middle of a poor, caucasian community. I'm not exaggerating when I tell you that every shift I worked, we had at least one call for a drug overdose.

The places that we would have to go for overdosed patients are places no one in their right mind would ever voluntarily step foot into. They were filthy, rundown, and smelled so awful you couldn't even breathe. I don't even want to know what type of rodents were hiding in the shadows of these places. It was actually so bad that our crew created a code word for when someone saw critters. If we were on a run and someone called out "disco", you better not stop moving your feet until we left the scene.

We didn't have an option, so run after run, shift after shift, we would respond to calls where people had overdosed. I can only speak for myself, but I quickly became numb to the people we were trying to save. My body went through the motions, but my mind was elsewhere. I started to feel anger burn throughout me, slowly at first, eventually building into a full-on rage. I know I shouldn't say this, but I started to not even care if some of these people woke up. We walked into places where the adults were overdosed on heroin and a toddler was walking around in a dirty diaper or an infant was crying on the couch. Those calls were the worst. A part of me didn't even want to give those people the Narcan, because according to how I felt, they didn't deserve a second chance at being parents. I was disgusted beyond belief. They weren't involved in a tragic car accident, fighting for their lives. They were chasing a high, with babies that needed to be fed and changed but had no other choice but to lie on a sofa and cry. I resented the people who chose to do this. Oh, and when we woke them up, do you think they were thankful that we just saved their lives? On the contrary. They were irate that we ruined their high. Sometimes they tried to fight us when they came to. A lot of the times, the drugs were laced with fentanyl or meth, giving the people superhuman strength. We would wake them up and give them a second chance at living, and they would cuss at us, try to fight us, or spit on us. There was no satisfaction in bringing them back.

This epidemic caused the highest body count I'd ever encountered. A lot of times we were able to wake them up, but many times, we weren't. I got so tired of seeing dead bodies with needles hanging out of their arms, or empty syringes in piles on the floor. We were all so burned out on responding to overdoses. I know that must sound heartless, but there is an actual term and condition for what I am describing to you called compassion fatigue. Compassion fatigue is essentially a physical and mental exhaustion that occurs in those who care for sick or traumatized patients for an extended period of time. The compassion fatigue made it extremely difficult for me to do my job. I started to dread going in to work. I dreaded when the tones would go off and we would have to respond to those types of calls. One of the only ways to overcome compassion fatigue is to take a break from stressful or traumatic exposures. For me, this meant taking a shift or two off of work. I could reset by getting out of the environment that was causing me copious amounts of stress. Unfortunately, as soon as I went back to work, I reverted right back to feeling the same lack of empathy. The duration of this didn't merely last days, weeks, or months, this would go on for a span of years.

I wish I could say that the memories from this time have faded and it doesn't bother me as much as it used to, but the truth is that those types of memories remain vivid and change who you are. You become a version of yourself that's so jaded, you can't go back to who you used to be before the job. There is only moving forward from here, and accepting that the tragic entries in the heroin diaries will forever be a part of my story.

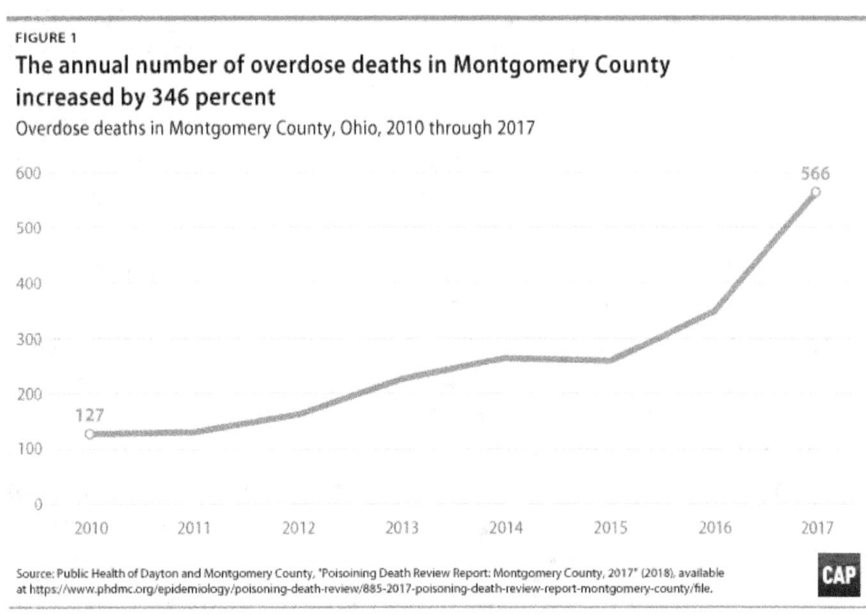

Graph courtesy of Public Health of Dayton and Montgomery County

14 – THE BOYS

"Of all the titles I've been privileged to have, 'Dad' has always been the best."
-Ken Norton

After going through some arduous stories, I'm delighted to talk about one of my favorite topics, my children. They have always been bright spots in my world, unknowingly shining on me when I felt lost in the shadows.

Lauren and I were ecstatic when she became pregnant with our first child. Much to the dismay of our families, we decided *not* to find out the gender of our baby. We discussed names that we liked for a girl and a boy. I didn't think much discussion would be necessary to pick out a boy's name. I am James Lawrence Burneka Jr; if we had a boy, he would obviously be James Lawrence Burneka III. Except there was discussion to be had, because Lauren shut that down. To be fair, I've never in my life gone by my given name of James, and neither has my dad. As a child I went by Jimmy, and now I go by Jim. Valerie, a friend of mine, suggested the name Jameson. She was on to something. I did like to drink the occasional Irish whiskey. We looked up the name, and the literal translation for Jameson is "son of James."

Lauren started having contractions June 15, 2013. We went to Southview hospital, ready to meet our baby! On June 16th, Jameson Liam Burneka came into the world. A lot of people gave us a hard time when we decided not to find out the gender, but the moment he was born was worth the nine months of not knowing. It was the most surreal feeling when the doctor announced, "It's a boy!" I was over the moon not only that we had a little boy, but that he and I shared a birthday. Yep, June 16th is my birthday as well! And as if the day didn't already contain enough excitement, June 16, 2013, was also Father's Day. Jameson really knew how to make a grand entrance.

Lauren and I were enamored with our perfect little boy. I felt as though nothing could take away the new-found joy we were experiencing. But the following day, something did. A doctor from Dayton Children's Hospital came to examine Jameson, and upon his examination, he heard a heart murmur. After doing some tests, it was confirmed that Jameson had a heart defect called ventricular septal defect (VSD). This was a fancy way of saying that he was born with a hole in his heart. I didn't want to believe that anything could be wrong with him—I mean, just look at him! He was the epitome of perfection.

I went from feeling on top of the world to completely deflated. My mind automatically went to worst-case scenarios. I guess my feelings were obvious, because the doctor attempted to lift my spirits. He brought me out of my spiral a little when he said, "He'll never be allowed in the army, but he still could be an Olympic athlete." I will never forget his words, because they gave me comfort at a time I felt helpless and defeated.

Jameson became a regular at the cardiologist's office. At first, he had to go biweekly, then graduated to monthly, and then every few months. We eventually made it to where we only have to visit annually. The older he gets, the smaller the hole becomes, and the chances of having to undergo a heart surgery decreases. Despite those odds, I still feel extremely anxious each year at this appointment.

I was reading a cancer research paper when something in the study jumped out and punched me straight in the gut. The study referenced a connection between the harmful carcinogens firefighters are surrounded by and their children being born with defects. I interviewed the researcher who conducted the study and asked her if there was a direct correlation between those exposed to harmful carcinogens and their offspring being born with defects. She said that they didn't see it enough to claim it was statistically significant, but there *was* an increase compared to the general population. I can't explain to you how sick I felt that somehow, there was a possibility that Jameson's heart defect was a result of harmful things I was exposed to at my job.

More research needs to be done in this specific area, but I believe it is reason enough for firefighters to take *every* precaution possible while at work. It is very possible that the carcinogens firefighters are exposed to at work can be passed down to their children. Our actions don't just affect us!

If you were to ask me, the only noticeable difference about Jameson's heart is that it's possibly made out of gold. That child has got the most gentle, kind heart I have ever seen. He is in all honors classes, as school comes easily to him. He isn't quite as much a natural in sports, but what he lacks in talent, he makes up for in hustle and effort. He works harder than most ten-year-olds I know to achieve the goals he sets for himself.

A couple years after Jameson was born, we found out that Lauren was pregnant again. We were so excited to be giving Jameson a sibling. This time around, we found out the gender of the baby—it was another boy! His original due date was none other than June 16th—the birthday that Jameson and I shared. Lauren couldn't believe it and was hoping that all three of us wouldn't have the same birthday! True to his personality, Logan Joseph Burneka entered the world on May 31st, a few weeks early, on his terms. Lauren and I both really liked the name Logan, and she wanted his middle name to be Joseph, after her father. My granddad and uncle are also named Joseph, so it is a significant name in our family.

I was nervous Logan would be born with a heart defect like Jameson, but he didn't have any issues at all. I can't tell you the relief I felt when Logan was born perfectly healthy. Logan is the yin to Jameson's yang. Whereas Jameson is quiet and shy, Logan is larger than life. The child doesn't know a stranger; he's friendly to everyone he encounters. He has a mop of curly blonde hair that compliments his wild personality. He is a beast at any sport he attempts. His abilities and instincts come naturally to him. He loves any and all animals and has a really close bond with my service dog, Bishop. Logan has the most contagious laughter, the kind you hear and find yourself randomly chuckling along with him.

Our two boys couldn't be any different, but what fun would it be to copy and paste all of your kids? Lauren wanted a third baby, hoping this time around it would be a girl. We both came from families with three siblings, so it seemed as though it would be the natural thing to do.

I understood she wanted a girl, but I kept having this nagging feeling that I wasn't going to live a long life. I didn't think it would be fair to bring another baby into a world that I wouldn't be in much longer. This was before my cancer diagnosis, and I had no real reason to question my mortality, but I couldn't shake the fear. Against Lauren's wishes, I had a vasectomy. In one procedure, I ruined her chances of ever having a little girl. She didn't understand my thought process, and truthfully, I didn't really understand it then either. All I knew was that I had such an intense fear of dying, that it overpowered all logical thinking. I couldn't be reasoned with.

I talked about this situation while I was at the Center of Excellence (a treatment and recovery facility I attended). I was told that the post-traumatic stress I had been experiencing was the main driver behind this decision. Normal people in a healthy frame of mind do not question their mortality, let alone allow the fear of dying determine big life decisions. I didn't know it at the time, but I was operating with a condition that prevented me from making sound decisions. I truly felt an overwhelming impending doom, like there was a time bomb inside of me, ready to explode at any given moment.

I feel badly about the way I handled the whole situation, and unfortunately, I can't take it back. I know this revelation is opening me up to the possibility of harsh criticism, but I share this because I want people to understand what it looks like living with post-traumatic stress. It wasn't really talked about then, so it wasn't on our radar. If you or your spouse are experiencing similar feelings, please seek help. It is not healthy, and there is help available for this condition.

My wife and children are my greatest joys here on earth. I will continue to fight in this battle for my mental health, because they deserve to have a healthy husband and father. Instead of counting down my days, I want to make the moments in each day count.

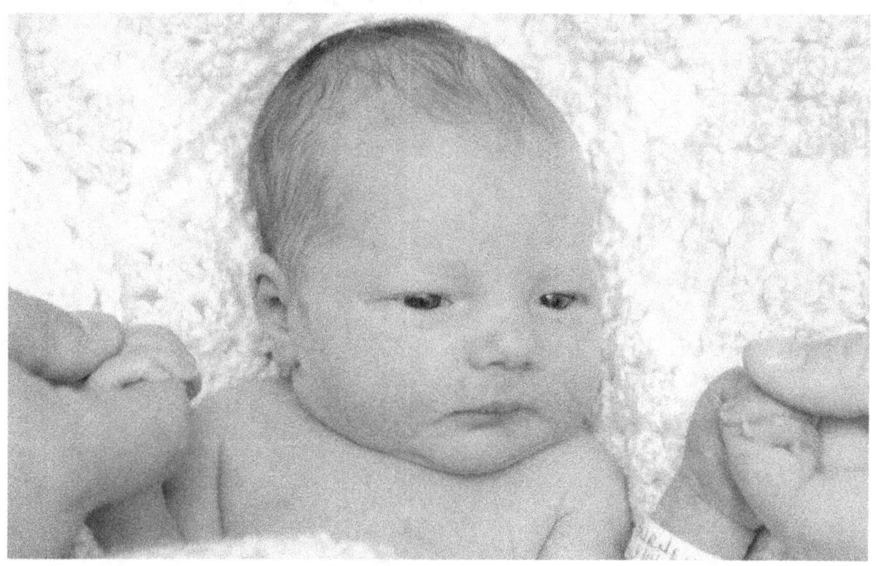

Baby Jameson

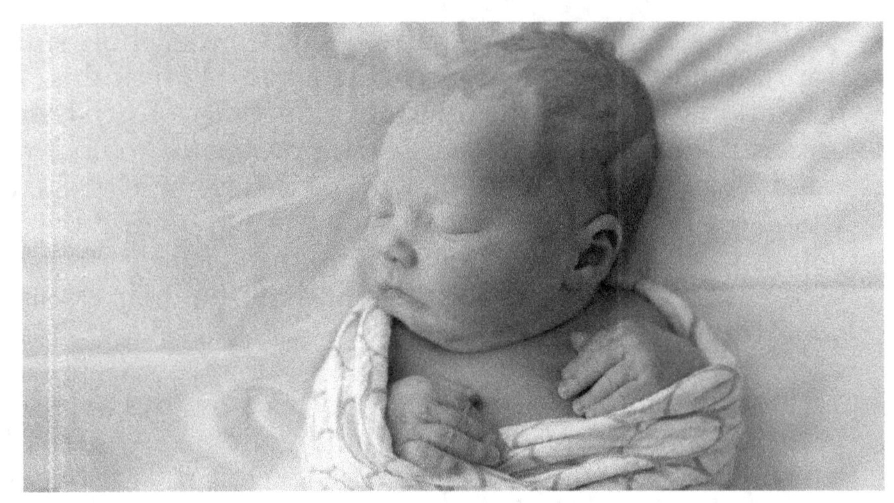

Baby Logan

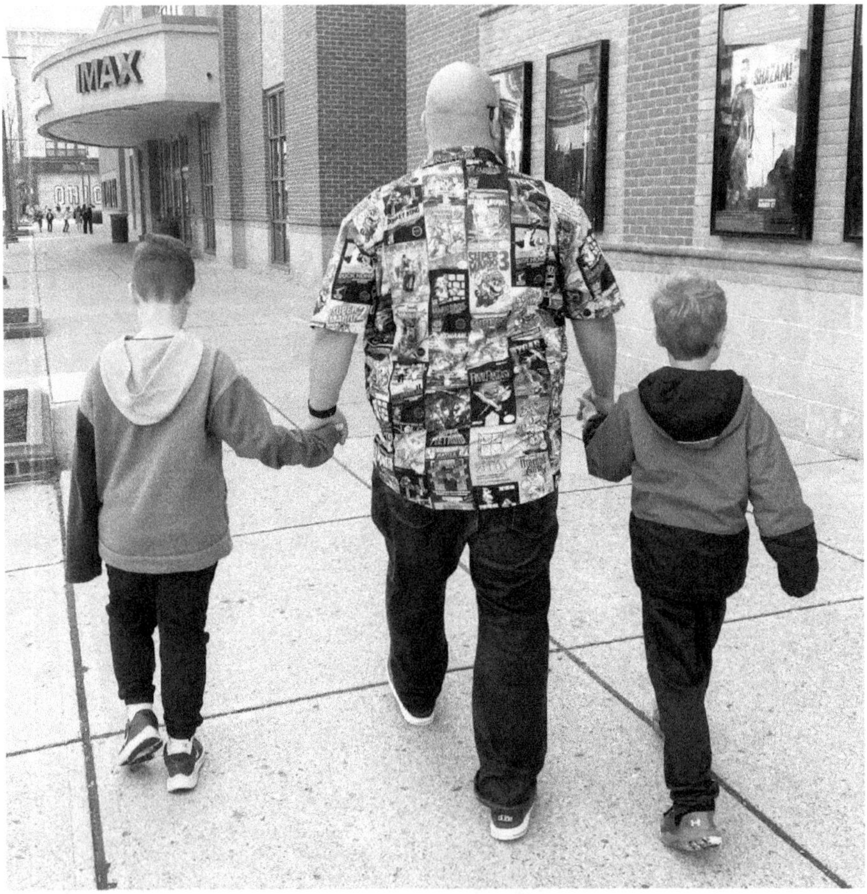

15 – ALMOST DOESN'T COUNT

*"If you fight you won't always win. But if you don't fight
you will always lose."*
-Bob Crow

After being on the job for about fifteen years, I decided if I was ever going to try for a promotion, now was the time. I was a husband and a father, and I wanted to be taken seriously. It was a big commitment preparing for the test, but I decided to take the plunge and try to get promoted to lieutenant. In Dayton, the exam to become a lieutenant is 125 multiple choice questions based off half a dozen commercial books, and half a dozen second drawer materials. Your chances of doing well on the test were high if you were good at memorization. I knew that just like in paramedic school and the academy, I was going to have to work incredibly hard to succeed.

It wasn't really the seat I would get to sit in or the pay raise that made me want to try to get promoted. It came down to the fact that I just wanted people to take me seriously. In Dayton, rank holds so much weight. If you were a firefighter and never climbed above that, you weren't taken seriously. Upper management rarely listened to what I had to say, and I thought that maybe if I had rank, they would have to listen to me.

I partnered up with some friends and spent the entire year studying. Everything that I did revolved around studying for the promotion exam. I leaned on my parents a lot to watch Jameson while Lauren worked so that I could study. They were happy to help us with him.

The friends that I studied with were confident in how well I knew the material. I knew that I didn't leave anything on the table. I put my all into studying for this exam. On the day of the exam, I was ready to move on up. Unfortunately, I didn't score as well as I should have on the test and wasn't promoted. There were twelve people who were promoted, and I was seventeenth on the list. I didn't fail and do terribly, but I didn't do well enough to make the cut.

I was devastated by my performance on the test. There was no good reason I didn't score higher. I knew the material and studied my butt off for an entire year. If I would've gotten promoted it would've been worth it, but now it just felt as if everything I'd done over the past year was in vain. I missed out on precious time with my son that I will never get back, for nothing. My parents and Lauren had to step in for me, for nothing. I felt so incredibly defeated.

About a year or so later, I decided to take the test again. However, it was going to be different this time. I wasn't willing to give up any more precious time with my family, so I didn't study like I had the first time around. I figured I would try again and see what happened, but I wasn't going to let my life revolve around a test. Unfortunately, the second test yielded the same results as the first one. I did not do well enough to be promoted to lieutenant for a second time. It was incredibly frustrating, but I also knew I didn't really put in the work. They say the third time's a charm, but I had no interest in going through the stress of taking the test a third time. As the years went by, I watched member after member become promoted, even though I had scored higher than them on the test. To their credit, they didn't give up like I did.

I tell you this story because I want to encourage you *not to give up*. If you fail a test, that's okay, take it again. Don't just give up and forget your goal. Although I'm disappointed I didn't pass the test, I'm not ashamed of my efforts. The other point of the story is that while position and rank carry a lot of value, they don't mean everything. Your position does *not* define who you are. It doesn't matter how high or low it may be, it doesn't define you as a person. Even as just a firefighter, I was still able to procure the wellness coordinator role. Eventually, people did take me seriously, sans *lieutenant* or *captain* before my name. Don't let failure stop you from reaching for your dreams and goals.

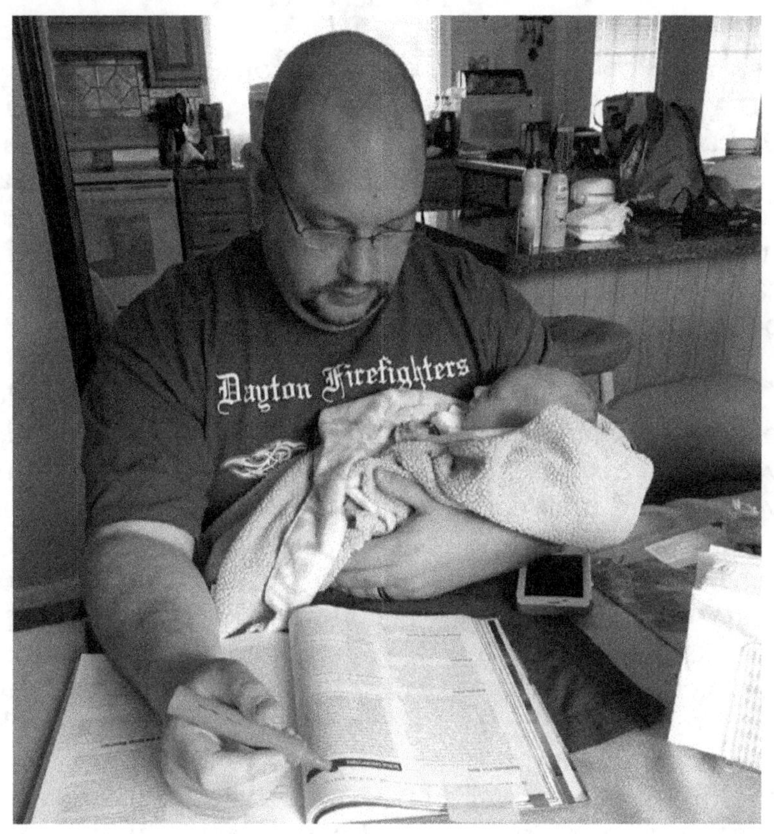

Logan and I putting in some study time

16 – RISING FROM THE ASHES

"I've failed over and over and that is why I succeed."
-Michael Jordan

After two failed attempts at promotion to lieutenant, I felt a sense of peace about moving on from that endeavor. However, I did not feel peace about losing my position with the FCSN. Whereas my pride took a hit from being fired from a volunteer position, my biggest frustration was that I felt as if I wasn't finished with the cancer awareness and prevention work I had started. If I'm being honest, I felt as though I'd just begun.

Lauren and I discussed different options I could pursue to continue my work in cancer awareness and prevention. This was such an interesting situation, because if you'd asked me years ago if this would be my passion, I would've laughed and called you crazy. But as I started learning about the threat of occupational cancer, it not only stirred me, but it wrecked me. When something wrecks you in a certain way, you have no choice but to take action. One thing I knew for certain was that I didn't want to be burnt by another organization I trusted. I knew the value I brought to the table, even if other people couldn't see it. I also had my two little boys to consider. Traveling took a new toll as I had to leave them behind. If I was going to be traveling without them, it really needed to be for something worthwhile.

We decided that there was only one option that made sense—starting my own company. I decided that I'd go to fire departments and take a deep dive into how they were handling firefighter cancer prevention. I'd observe how they function in the firehouse as well as on scene, and post-call. I'd then compare their protocols and actions based upon the current best practices and cancer initiatives. Once I gathered all of the data and information, I'd write it all down in a comprehensive report. In the report I'd state the current practice, the recommended changes they could implement, and the estimated cost to put the changes in place. I scored each area of the department, presenting a clear picture of the risks within their station, and practical ways to minimize or eliminate them.

The first station I did was my own. This was not a paid project, but a passion project. I had the opportunity to do this as I was on light-duty, recovering from an ACL reconstructive surgery. After understanding the risk of cancer firefighters face, I had to take action. Even if it wasn't groundbreaking, it was a start to a healthier and longer life for my crew.

During my time with FCSN, I created a sign that read, "No Fire Gear Beyond This Point," and hung it on the doors going into the living quarters to make sure we don't bring carcinogens into our living areas. Variations of that sign are now used universally in stations. That sign alone was proof that tiny changes can have large impacts. Even if it was just a small station here or there, I knew that I could make a difference.

The Firefighter Cancer Consultants was born, and I was really excited about my new company. I embraced the opportunity to help departments become progressive in the battle against cancer. I started promoting my company, trying to drum up some business, and little by little I started picking up momentum and getting work.

For a few years, I would work my normal shift and travel to various departments on my days off to do my consulting work. Then the City of Dayton caught wind of what I was doing, and like they do best, they tried to squash the little guy. They told me that per the city charter, I was not allowed to have my side company and needed to cease and desist.

By now I realized that to the city, I wasn't Jim Burneka, founder of Firefighter Cancer Consultants. I wasn't Jim Burneka, son, husband, brother, and father. I was simply a number, disposable and easily replaceable. I knew I had to fight back, so I hired an attorney to keep my company. It was a colossal waste of time and money for myself, as well as the City of Dayton. The city's brilliant solution was for me to put my business in my wife's name.

In the end, I got to keep my (now Lauren's) company, as I wasn't doing anything that breached my contract. My soul was getting weary, but my backbone stronger. I was no longer a simple pawn, I was a voice, and I wouldn't allow them to silence me any longer.

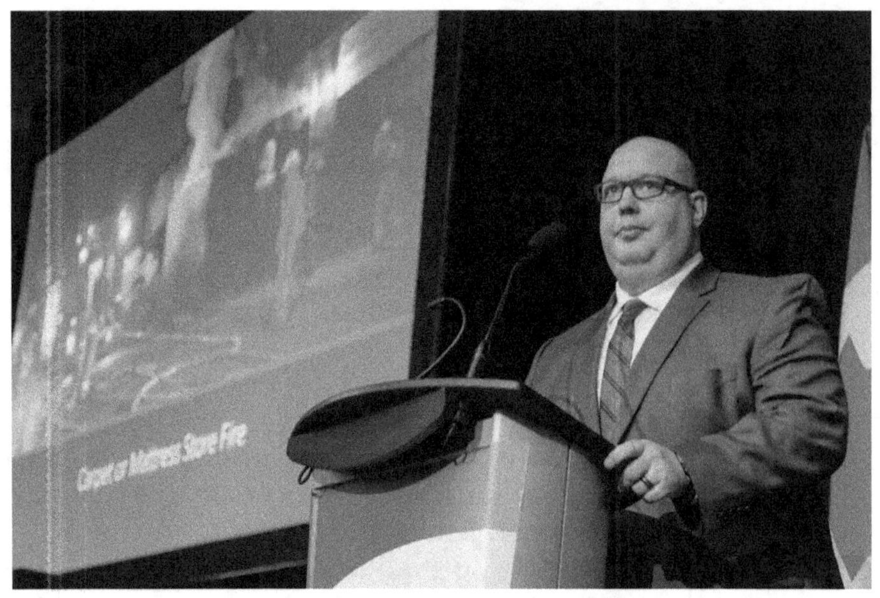

Speaking at the Canadian Fire Chiefs Conference

17 – HEARING LOSS

"What?"
-Jim Burneka

I had found my voice, but I began to notice that I was having difficulty hearing when I was in a noisy environment. For example, if I was on the back of the engine, I couldn't hear what my crew was saying. However, when I was talking to someone in a quiet environment, I could hear them just fine. It didn't really make sense to me. When it was time for my annual physical, I was certain that there would be some red flags on my hearing test. Much to my surprise, my test came back completely normal. This would go on for a few years. I was getting really frustrated. My hearing tests were coming back normal, but my hearing was getting progressively worse.

Finally, I took a hearing test and the doctor came back in and announced, "Everything looks good!" I told him that everything was in fact *not* good. Something was wrong with my hearing. He said that there are only two hospitals in our state that can do a more thorough evaluation. I called both places, and I made an appointment with the hospital with the shortest waiting period, which was thirteen months.

Meanwhile, when I was on the medic or engine, I really struggled to hear what was going on. This was a massive safety risk in a profession like mine. Being in a fire or on scene, it is imperative I am able to hear commands and what my crew is saying. The thirteen months of waiting seemed impossibly long, as I was desperate for someone to pinpoint what was wrong with my hearing. I became proficient at reading lips during this time and began avoiding crowded, noisy environments.

Finally on June 7th, 2017, I went to see Dr. Whitelaw at the Ohio State Hearing and Language Center. Her tests were nothing like the quick tests I had done at my annual exams. I sat in a booth for a good forty-five minutes doing various tests. She also did a thorough exam of the inside of my ears, taking measurements and examining every aspect of them. It was a very in-depth evaluation.

When Dr. Whitelaw was finished, she confirmed what I had been saying for years. I passed every hearing test, but I had failed the background hearing tests miserably. This meant that if I was in a quiet environment, I could hear everything fine. But put me in a place where there is a lot of noise in the background, I can't really hear anything. The readings in my ears also showed that my follicles were dead. She said that her findings from my exam were consistent with signs of carbon monoxide poisoning. There were a lot of times early in my career when I didn't wear my mask and was exposed to high amounts of carbon monoxide. It was highly likely that my job had cost me a part of my hearing.

I was relieved that someone finally validated the hearing loss I had been experiencing. Unfortunately, the damage done to my hearing was not reversible. There were no procedures that could fix it. The only viable option would be to get hearing aids. You might be thinking, "That's great Jim. It will solve your problems." The problem with hearing aids is that they are extremely expensive. I had no idea how I'd ever be able to afford them.

I borrowed some hearing aids from Dr. Whitelaw's office, but that was only a short-term solution. I was telling a friend about what was going on with my hearing, and he said that he was able to get his hearing aids paid for through an agency called Opportunities for Ohioans with Disabilities (OOD). He put me in touch with them, and they covered my hearing aids in full. I was so relieved and thankful. Finally, I would be able to hear again!

The more people I talked to about my hearing loss, the more people admitted they'd been suffering from the same exact thing. When the doctors told them they passed the hearing test, they accepted it and moved on. I have learned throughout the years that if you don't advocate for yourself, *no one* will. Sometimes you have to stand up to people and have hard conversations to be able to receive the help you need. I was able to point these people to Dr. Whitelaw, and if they needed hearing aids (in most cases they did), I put them in contact with OOD. After learning that carbon monoxide poisoning was likely the cause of my hearing loss, it wasn't surprising that other firefighters were dealing with the same thing. Although this more than likely occurred during our job, it was too hard to prove to make a workers compensation case out of it.

I am a huge advocate for firefighters wearing their personal protective equipment (PPE) during fires and overhaul, to prevent breathing in carcinogens, but also to prevent suffering from carbon monoxide poisoning. Back when I first started twenty-two years ago, we didn't know what we didn't know. Now with all of the research and findings that have come to light, there's no reason for any firefighter to not be wearing their protective equipment. I'm begging people to learn from my mistakes!

My wife would be the first to tell you that I don't always listen, but at least now I could hear.

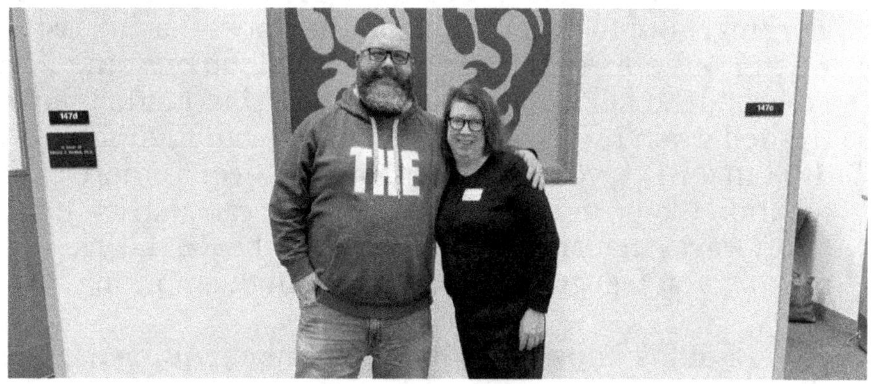

Dr. Whitelaw and I at the Ohio State University Speech and Hearing Clinic

18 – SLEEPY TIME

"Early to bed and early to rise makes a man healthy, wealthy, and wise."
Benjamin Franklin

Sometimes it seemed as if once I solved one problem, another one immediately emerged. I had taken care of my hearing problem, only to be struggling with sleep. The life of a firefighter is complicated in regard to sleeping. Shift work is very difficult because there is no guarantee you will get any sleep. A lot of the time, even if it's a slow night at work, falling asleep is hard because you're anticipating the tones going off at any given moment. If you do catch a run in the middle of the night, it's hard to get your body back into a calm state to be able to relax and go to sleep.

My lack of sleep was very problematic, not just when I was on shift. The issues carried over into my home life, and I struggled to maintain a good night's sleep. Even when I slept for a good number of hours, I still felt depleted when I woke up.

I went to the doctor and was prescribed Ambien as a sleeping aid. Obviously, I could not take this when I was working, but I took it at home in the hopes that at least when I was off work, I'd be able to catch up on some sleep. I'd be able to fall asleep taking Ambien, but I didn't feel refreshed when I woke up. After looking into it, Ambien is a drug that helps you fall asleep, but the sleep is more of a sedation than true sleep. The medicine can restrict the brain waves that are produced during the REM cycle, making you feel groggy and drowsy in the morning.

I didn't know this when I was taking Ambien, and I slightly abused the medication. Once I was on a red-eye from California to Ohio, and I took it so that I could fall asleep on the flight. The problem with this was that it wasn't a direct flight. A flight attendant had to wake me up so that I could exit the plane, and I stumbled down the boarding bridge and sat down at a random gate. Thankfully, a retired Dayton firefighter was flying home from somewhere and saw me sitting there asleep. He woke me up to say hi, and proceeded to walk with me to our gate. (we were going on the same flight home.) He could tell then I was out of it and kept an eye on me until we landed. After that experience, I never took another Ambien.

I knew there had to be a reason sleep evaded me, so I scheduled a sleep study. They hooked me up to a ton of wires and sensors at the sleep doctors' office, and someone monitored me while I slept. It was evident to them during the study that I had sleep apnea. It recorded my breath pausing about fifty times in an hour. That is a significantly high number! They gave me a continuous positive airway pressure (CPAP) machine, and I use it every night when I sleep. With this machine my body is able to fall into a deep sleep. Even if I sleep for fewer hours than before, I wake up feeling more refreshed, because I'm getting a much better quality of sleep.

It's much easier to get a sleep study done now versus years ago when I had mine done. If you have symptoms of sleep apnea such as excessive, loud snoring or just waking up feeling tired, you might want to look into doing a sleep study. They can order them for you to do in the comfort of your own home. There are just a few pieces of equipment involved, such as a nasal cannula, a pulse oximeter, and a chest strap. It's nothing like what I had to do when I had my study done.

Sleep apnea runs rampant among people in the fire industry. One study showed that out of 70,000 firefighters, nearly 40% suffer from a sleep-related issue, such as insomnia, sleep apnea, or work shift disorder. Firefighters need to make sleep a priority. One way they can do this is to not schedule anything for a few hours after they get off of shift, so that they can take a nap.

Sleep is the foundation of all things wellness. Firefighters (as well as everyone else) must prioritize getting quality sleep. A lot of times when we get busy, sleep is the first thing we cut out in order to fit more things into our day. Realistically, sleep is the last thing we should cut out. Please try to take the necessary measures to ensure you are getting quality sleep at night.

Now that I was getting good, quality sleep, I started dreaming again. I realized that I could easily turn one of my dreams into reality.

19 – GO THE DISTANCE

"We just don't recognize life's most significant moments while they're happening. Back then I thought, "Well, there'll be other days." I didn't realize that was the only day."
-Dr. Archibald "Moonlight" Graham – Field of Dreams

In my younger years, I completed my bucket list of visiting all thirty Major League Baseball parks. Although I was able to check that off my list, there was still one prominent baseball field I had yet to visit that I wanted to see—the Field of Dreams in Iowa.

Growing up, my dad and I watched the *Field of Dreams* movie, and although he had seen it before, he still got lost in the magic of it each time we watched it. I dreamed of visiting that field, and I knew that if I was going to take that trip, it wouldn't be complete unless my dad came with me.

I told my dad to pack his clothes, that we were going on a five-day road trip! I didn't tell him where the final destination of our trip would be, and he was okay with being surprised. I rented a car and we started to head west. I didn't plan out our trip with a lot of details. I just figured when I got tired of driving, we'd find a hotel and crash for the night. That method would stress out a lot of people, but it worked for us. We went at our own pace, stopping for food and to stretch our legs without having any time constraints. One night, we stumbled upon an awesome jazz festival in Peoria, Illinois. My dad loves jazz music, so I couldn't have planned it any better. They had great food at this festival, and we both enjoyed ourselves. We also stopped by the *American Pickers* building and took our time just looking around.

By this point my dad had figured out where we were heading, but I didn't mind that it wasn't a big surprise. I had bought tickets to a "ghost game," which is a baseball game where players dress up and emerge from the corn and onto the field to play a game. It ended up canceled due to rain. I wasn't too disappointed the ghost game was cancelled, as that was just the icing on the cake. The real treat was getting to actually walk on the iconic Field of Dreams baseball field. Because it had been raining, it wasn't crowded at all. My dad and I soaked in the magic and nostalgia that the field held, both of us transported into a place of wonder and joy. In a surreal moment, we played catch in the outfield. We even walked through the cornfield onto the outfield and quoted lines from the movie such as, "Is this Heaven? No, it's Iowa." Yes, it's cheesy, but if you go there, you've got to do that.

Getting to experience the Field of Dreams with my dad was even better than I'd anticipated. We caught a Brewers vs. Cubs game in Milwaukee on the way home, and it was the perfect ending to our road trip. Yes, the *Field of Dreams* movie is about baseball, but also redemption. Fitting, as this trip turned out to be redemptive within our relationship. I'm forever grateful we bit the bullet and decided to go the distance.

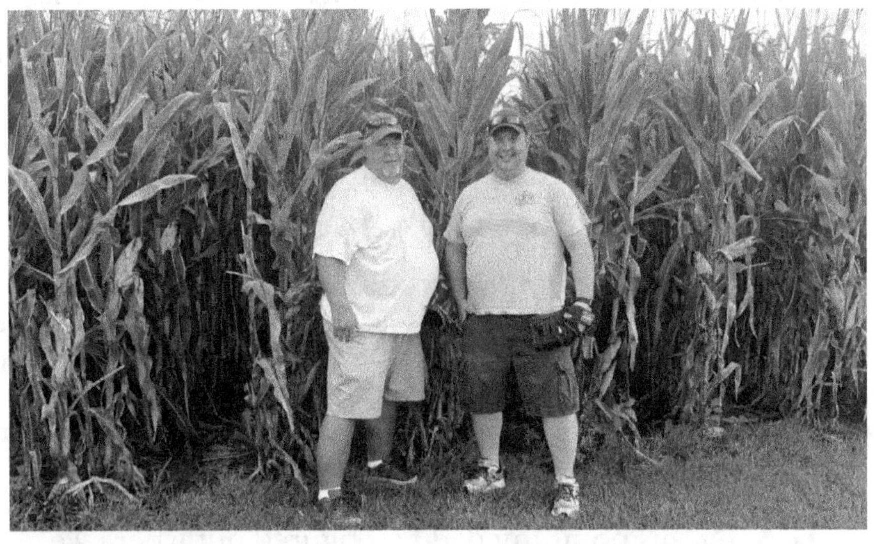

Dad & I at the Field of Dreams

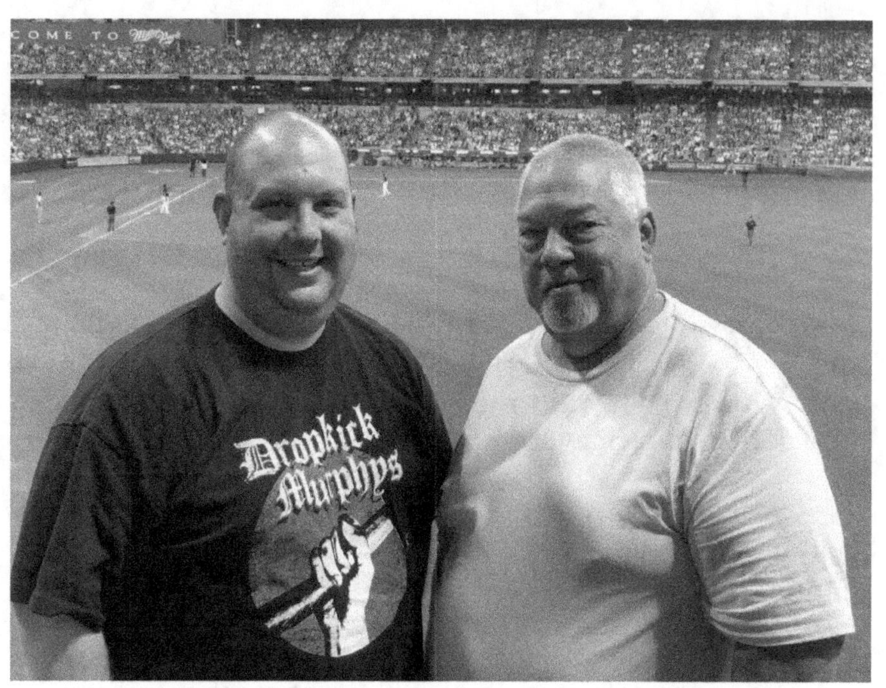

Catching a Cubs vs Brewers game in Milwaukee

20 – THE EXOTIC CONFERENCE

"Sometimes you want to go, where everybody knows your name, and they're always glad you came. You want to be where you can see, our troubles are all the same; you want to be where everybody knows your name."
-Cheers

My dad and I got completely caught up in the nostalgia at the enchanted Field of Dreams in Iowa. Now it was time to make some magic happen back home in Beavercreek, Ohio.

I was approached by Nick Magoteaux in early 2017 about a Firefighters Health and Wellness Conference he wanted to start. Nick is the founder of Brothers Helping Brothers, an organization that helps small and rural fire departments acquire the lifesaving tools and equipment they need to safely and properly execute their job duties. Nick clearly has a heart for helping others, especially the underprivileged.

Nick's idea for a local health and wellness conference was brilliant. He told me the vision he had for the conference, as well the speakers he was hoping to bring in. I told him that the speakers he wanted to pursue were great, but certain guys wouldn't want to be around other guys. It was a little hard to navigate the personal dynamics between the speakers. He couldn't believe the petty politics involved in planning the conference. I volunteered to help him organize the event, as well as do the cancer-awareness portion of it. Nick handled the behavior wellness portion of it. For the first conference, the cancer portion was a major focus point, with snippets of behavioral health thrown in. Years later, we have adjusted the itinerary to where behavioral health is the main focus of the event. Cancer awareness is still important, but we realized how prominent mental health issues are, and pivoted to cover a big portion of that topic.

Nick and I made a great team, and through planning the conference, we became good friends. We discovered that we had a great balance, as he was gifted in handling all of the behind-the-scenes aspects of planning, and I was better at coordinating the front-of-house aspects. He's great at taking care of the website and registration and paperwork side of things. I am more comfortable setting up the speakers and making sure they have what they need and are good to go.

The big firefighter conferences are in desirable locations with beautiful weather, such as Florida, California, or Las Vegas. The tickets to attend these conferences typically run several hundred dollars, not including food and hotel accommodations. Nick's vision was a smaller, more intimate conference that was affordable to everyone. We could do it in our hometown of Beavercreek, Ohio, a small suburb of Dayton. We knew that we couldn't compete with the big guys, but we could still put together a very informative and impactful conference. We started to refer to the location of our conference as "Exotic Beavercreek, Ohio." We even created a logo with a beaver wearing sunglasses, and the words "Exotic Beavercreek, Ohio" surrounding the beaver. We hold our conference in October, and the weather is anything but tropical in Ohio in the fall. There is literally nothing exotic about Beavercreek, Ohio, but it's a perfect depiction of how we approach planning our conference. It's a little more lighthearted, with a theme each year and a more intimate setting. Some of the themes we've had include Vegas, Hollywood, and in the near future, wrestling. We obtained amazing sponsors, so we're able to get incredible speakers to join our panel while keeping the cost of tickets to attend down to a mere seventy-five dollars for three days of training. We firmly believe that everyone should have the opportunity to enhance their training without going broke.

This year, we're coming up on our sixth conference, and it's an event that I think will continue to grow with time. We work really hard to put on a conference that firefighters will benefit from, and we've realized that we can make a significant impact without being the biggest and best. I hope to continue our Firefighters Health and Wellness Conference for many years to come.

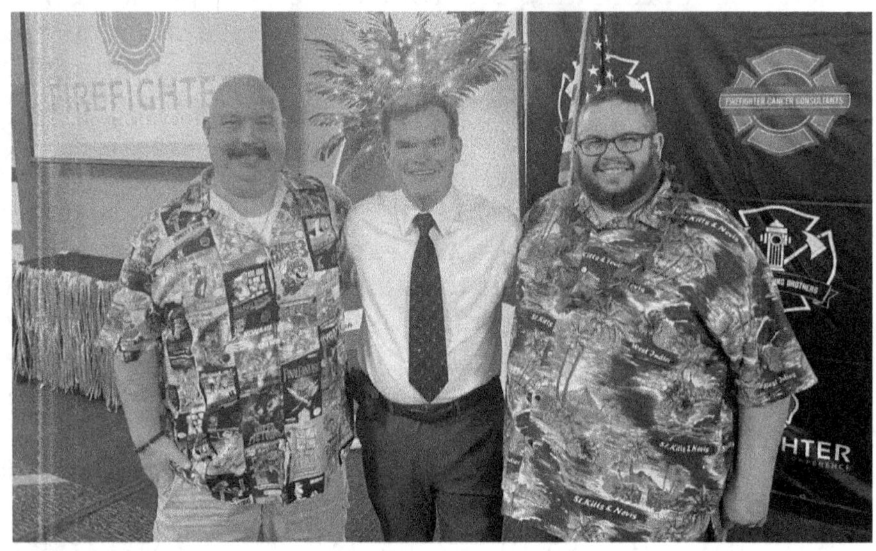

Me, Pat Kenny & Nick Magoteaux at our conference

21 – BOBBY

"I don't say goodbye anymore, I say see ya later."
-Bobby Hetzer

For someone who dove headfirst into firefighter health and wellness, I often ignored what I preached, especially when it came to dealing with big emotions. This will become apparent later in this story as I inwardly struggled with processing grief.

I first met Bobby early on in my career. He introduced himself to me and told me he knew my extended family. He laughed at me and told me there was no way I was a Burneka, because I was too small and didn't have knee problems. (He'd be happy to know that three knee surgeries later and quite a few pounds heavier, I have grown into my name.)

Bobby was beloved by everyone. He was an incredible cook at the firehouse and the best storyteller. He would capture your attention with a story and have you on the edge of your seat, crying laughing at the end of it. Bobby was a huge Bengals fan and kept binders full of players and potential recruits' stats. He loved to go to their games. His signature look consisted of never buttoning his top shirt button, letting a little chest hair fly around. Bobby was the type of guy that everyone genuinely enjoyed being around.

He worked a ton of overtime; so much so that when he retired, it was with the pension of a district chief. Bobby was forced to retire earlier than he wanted to due to neck issues. He moved to Nashville, but we still kept in touch. I would continue to see him at Bengals games.

Bobby got sick with pancreatic cancer. If you aren't familiar with it, pancreatic cancer is a really tough cancer to have. His spirits remained high, despite living with a painful cancer. Bobby ended up with an infection that turned septic. I received word that he wasn't doing well and was planning on leaving to see him right after my shift ended. The sepsis moved faster than my shift, and before I even finished working, he had passed away.

I helped plan a funeral for him, including all of the firefighter bells and whistles, since the cancer had been occupational. His son, Bronson, gave the eulogy at his funeral, and to this day, it's the best eulogy I've ever heard. He perfectly captured the essence of who his dad was, and expressed it with grace and humor. He definitely received the gift of storytelling from his dad. One story in particular he told stuck with me. He talked about him and his dad driving in the car with the top down, breeze whipping his chest hair around, and Bon Jovi turned up. Bobby was loudly singing along, messing up the lyrics. Bronson told him that he wasn't singing the right words, and Bobby replied, "Well, Jon really messed that up, didn't he?" If you had the pleasure of knowing Bobby, you could envision this entire story and would be able to hear the whole exchange.

About a year after his death, there was an annual ceremony at the International Association of Fire Fighters (IAFF) Fallen Firefighter's Memorial in Colorado Springs. I was going to attend the ceremony and present an IAFF flag to Bobby's widow, Michelle. These ceremonies are a big deal, and there were rehearsals for three mornings before the actual ceremony took place. I had to prepare something to say to Michelle as I presented the flag to her. I wanted to make sure I got it right, so I called my buddy, Scott, who'd previously been in one of these ceremonies, and asked for his advice. He told me to figure out what I wanted to say and rehearse it over and over until I didn't even have to think about what I was going to say. I took his advice and practiced what I wanted to tell Michelle until I memorized it and could comfortably express my condolences.

When it came time for the ceremony, I was extremely nervous. Out of over 200 people, my assigned seat was next to a friend of mine, Paul Jacques. I knew that wasn't a coincidence and was grateful to be sitting next to a friend. It definitely eased my nerves. When it was my turn to stand up and present the flag to Michelle, I don't remember exactly what I said, but I remember that I said it just the way I'd practiced.

After I gave Michelle the flag, I started crying, feeling myself crumble inside. All of the honor guards that had given flags were dismissed, and we were to walk down a path that was lined with pipers and drummers on each side of the walkway. This ceremony was for fallen firefighters throughout the entire U.S. as well as Canada, so you can imagine what a special and large production this was. The line of pipers and drummers went on and on, farther than I could see. It was pretty incredible to be a part of the commemoration. It was the biggest honor to have participated in the ceremony; however, I never wanted to do it again. Sometimes honor comes with a price. This time, the cost was deep anguish, buried into the crevices of my heart.

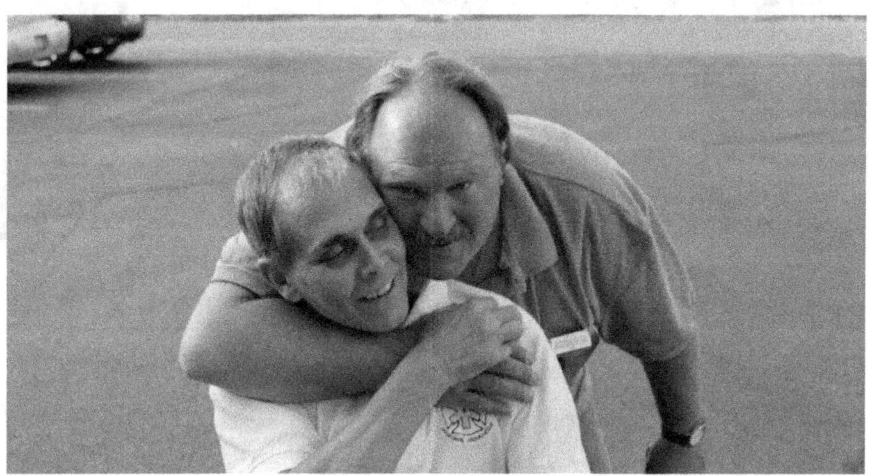

Bobby and Rod

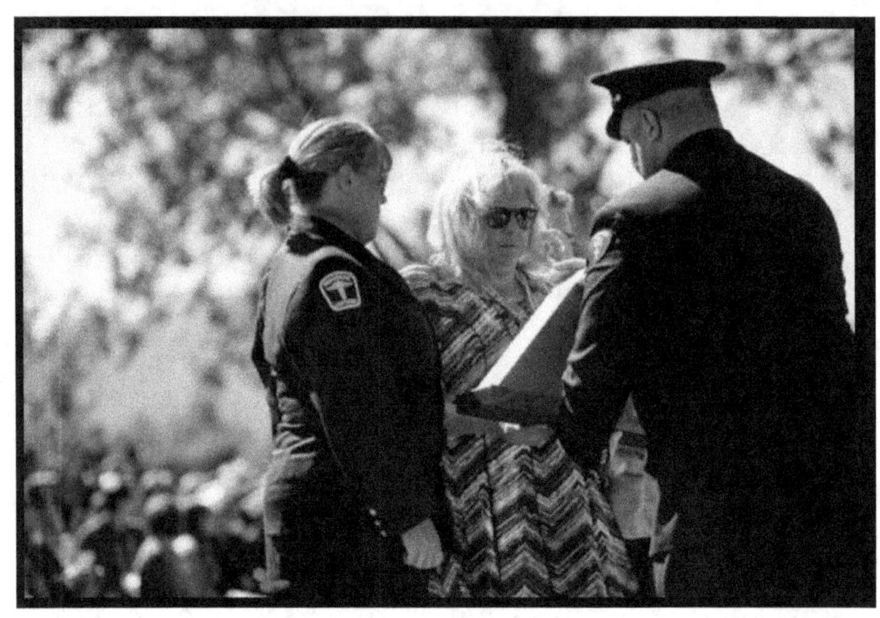

Giving Michelle Hetzer an IAFF flag

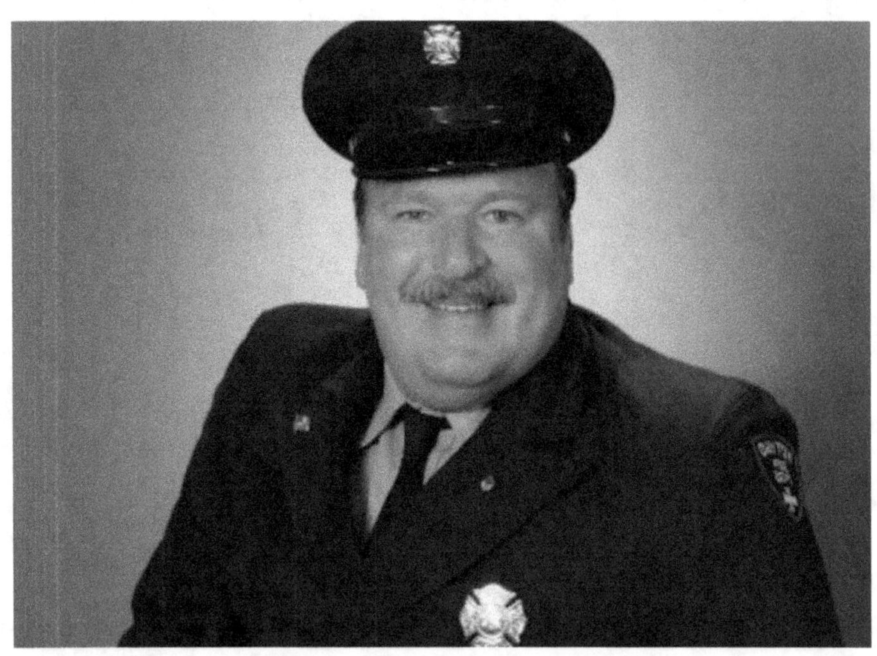

Robert "Bobby" Hetzer
10/30/1961 - 10/26/2018

22 – DR. DONNIE

"Don't get so busy making a living that you forget to make a life."
-Dolly Parton

I desperately wanted to help anyone that was in distress, as well as be present for my family. There never seemed to be enough hours in the day to accomplish everything I felt I needed to do. If I was thriving at work, I was dropping the ball at home. If I was consumed with family things, I was failing at the various roles I held at work. *Something* had to give, but I didn't know *what.*

I was introduced to Dr. Donnie Hutchinson when he taught a class at the union hall on how to achieve a healthy work-life balance. Dr. Donnie is a speaker, author, and online coach who works with first responders on various self-care and work-life strategies to help them be effective at their jobs as well as in their homes.

I was thankful I was able to sit in his class, as I was struggling with achieving a good work-life balance. My plate was full at the time, trying to juggle my family, work, union duties, etcetera. I was spread too thin, and wasn't maintaining a good balance between my job and my family.

I had the privilege of speaking with Dr. Donnie after his class. He made a lot of sense and gave a lot of practical applications to help me find a balance. I also read his book, *Lead With Balance.* Between his class and his book, I learned a lot from Dr. Donnie.

I'm going to share a few highlights I think would be beneficial to anyone reading this book. One great takeaway is that every time you say *yes* to something, you are saying *no* to something else. If you say *yes* to working overtime, you may be saying *no* to going to your kids' soccer game. You get the gist of it. Another highlight is to think about when your kids are grown—are they ever going to tell you that they're glad you worked so much? Spoiler alert, probably not. Work-life-balance is all about following through with your true priorities in life.

One exercise that Dr. Donnie did with us that was super effective was to have us close our eyes while he played Kenny Chesney's song "Don't Blink." If you haven't heard the song, it's a beautiful song that reflects on how fast life flies by, and reminds the listener to cherish every moment we're granted here on earth. After listening to the song, he asked us what we thought about while we were listening. Most people thought about their spouse or children. He asked if anyone thought about work throughout the song. The answer is always *no*. While work is something you have to *do*, it is not *who you are*. Work isn't everything.

It's a safe assumption that most first responders put others before themselves. Their actions show this sentiment each time they put on their gear or place a badge over their chest. They run into dangerous situations with the goal of helping people. Often times they're putting themselves *in* very harmful situations to get citizens *out* of them. We must take the time to care for ourselves, or we won't be able to help others. You know the saying, no one can pour from an empty cup.

Later in my career when I became plagued with terror from a previous run, I'd recognize that I needed to get ahold of my fear, as it was spilling over into work and home. I realized that when things were off-kilter in one place, it directly affected the other. Recognizing the problem was one thing, getting help and solving the problem was another.

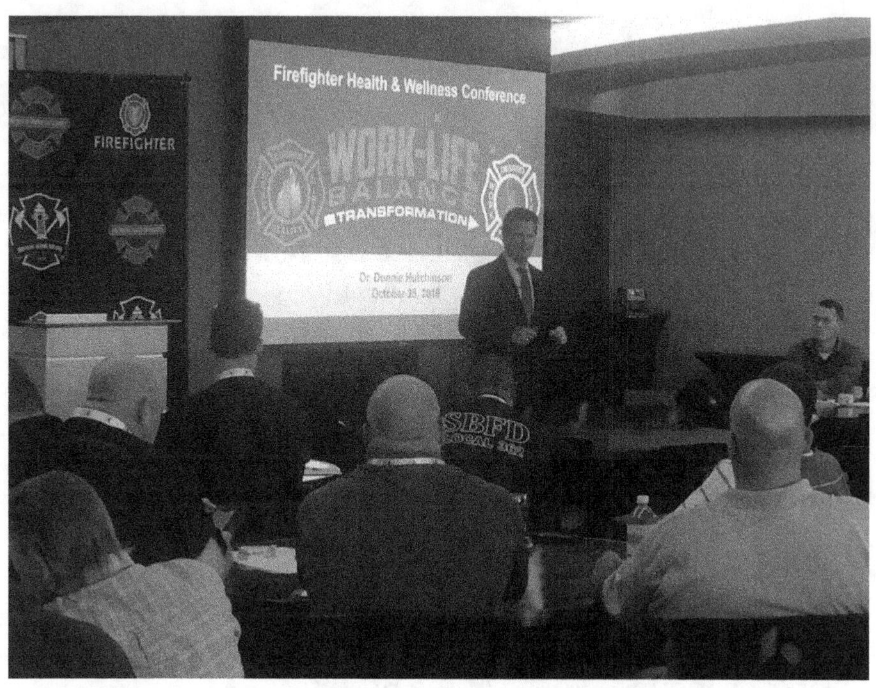

Dr. Donnie teaching Work-Life-Balance at our 2nd Annual FF Health & Wellness Conference

23 – THE DROWNING

"There's no tragedy in life like the death of a child. Things never get back to the way they were."
-Dwight D. Eisenhower

There is a delicate balance between work and home-life, as well as being able to function on the job while maintaining a healthy mental state. There's a learning curve to this balance, and it took being involved in deeply traumatic situations for me to come to this realization. Within my first five years on the job, we were dispatched to a drowning. Running lights and sirens, we sped to the scene. Upon our arrival, we encountered a little girl, no more than three years old, face down in a pond. She wasn't conscious or breathing. We got her loaded into the medic, frantically trying to bring her back to life. We transported her to the hospital as fast as we could. She was later pronounced dead at the hospital.

We were all really upset that we weren't able to save her. She still had her whole life ahead of her. We gave it our all trying to get her tiny heart beating again, but we didn't succeed. It really sucked. Although we were all struggling over the loss, we didn't talk about it. I know it sounds inhumane, but we went back to the station and prepared for our next run. Just because we didn't talk about it, it doesn't mean that it didn't bother us. It simply wasn't the culture to come back to the station and cry over runs. *No one* could endure our job if we did that. We quickly developed calluses around our hearts—not to be cruel, but to survive.

I didn't really think about that run over the years, until about a decade later. All of the sudden, I began reliving this call, every day. I really couldn't tell you why this call began to haunt me. The details from it would jolt me out of my sleep, keeping me awake all night. I was afraid to close my eyes, because I didn't want to go back to that nightmare. It was like a video on loop, playing over and over again. I had moved back to Station 15's and would pass the house where the drowning occurred several times throughout my shift. It shook me each time we passed the house, but I never said a word about it to anyone. I suffered silently, too ashamed to ask for help.

Finally, I'd reached a point of exhaustion that I could no longer sustain. I called a trusted clinician I had previously worked with and explained to her what I'd been experiencing. She told me that she thought I would benefit from Eye Movement Desensitization and Reprocessing (EMDR) therapy. This was a type of therapy that is used to work through traumatic experiences. It helps reprocess the memories, thus reducing the stress associated with the traumatic event. This is a common therapy for treating people who suffer from post-traumatic stress (PTS).

The best, non-medical way I can explain EMDR is for you to picture your brain as a filing cabinet. Every memory you have should go into a file folder within that cabinet. A memory from a traumatic incident doesn't get put into a folder; or the filing cabinet, for that matter. Envision it sitting on top of the filing cabinet. EMDR helps to place the memory back inside the filing cabinet, and into the proper folder.

It helps to repair the mental injury that was sustained, and although it doesn't erase the memory, the associated feelings that come along with it are much more manageable. They no longer overtake you and all of your emotions.

I had to talk about the event in great detail with my clinician, but I had a few gaps in my memory. I felt foolish, but I had to call the other guys that went on the run with me and ask them to fill in the blanks for me. The hardest phone call for me to make regarding this was to my lieutenant who was on that call. He was a seasoned officer; he had witnessed truly horrific events. He was as tough as nails and didn't show emotions. I was sure he would ridicule me for struggling with this call ten years after it happened. So, imagine my surprise when I called him and he was completely receptive to what I was saying. He assured me that I wasn't the first to reach out to him about runs we'd been on, and that it's not uncommon for things to come up years after the event occurred. He gravely told me that this job will take a toll on everyone; *no one* sees what we see and comes out unscathed.

In order to do this therapy, you have to sit and talk about the event with your clinician, holding little vibrating paddles as you do so. It is obviously not fun or enjoyable to talk about an event that has damaged you, but you must embrace it to get to the other side. Sometimes it only takes one session to properly reprocess the memory. Other times it could take half a dozen sessions. It took me four sessions to properly reprocess the drowning memory.

I am sharing this story, because EMDR is a powerful, effective tool for first responders. There is absolutely no shame in asking for help or going through this type of therapy. It's a safe and effective way to process trauma. I've gone through EMDR several times, the end result successful each time. I recommended this type of therapy to members who were suffering from traumatic events when I was in my wellness coordinator role. I urge you not to wait until the trauma becomes unbearable for you to carry; lay it down and allow someone to help you.

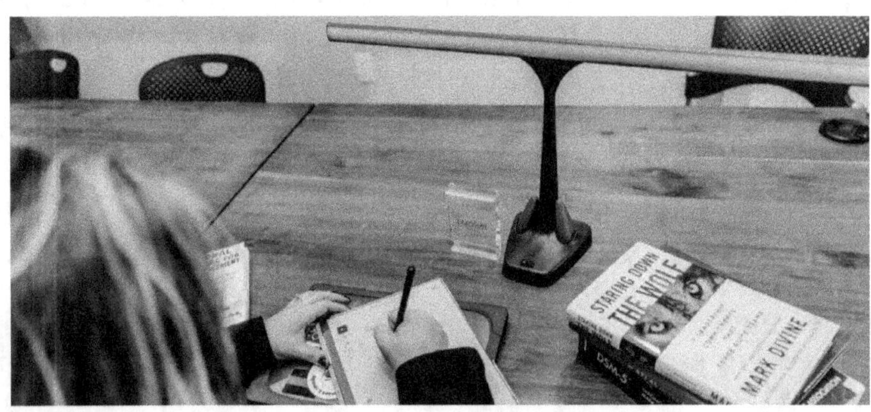

Alison and her EMDR light bar

24 – A SERIOUSLY TWISTED WEEKEND

"We will never be defined by tragedy but, instead, by how we respond to it."
-Kevin Brady

Firefighters are truly multifaceted, responding to a vast range of calls. Most of the calls didn't surprise me, but having to work at a hate rally was one gig I never saw coming. The Honorable Sacred Knights of the Ku Klux Klan (HSK) applied to hold a rally in downtown Dayton. The HSK are based out of Indiana, and they're a white supremacist group that spreads messages of hate and division.

Clearly no one thought this was a good idea or wanted the HSK to come to town. However, the HSK threatened to sue the City of Dayton if their application wasn't approved, under the guise it prohibited their constitutional right to freedom of speech. The city didn't really have another option but to allow them to come.

In May of 2019, the city prepared for the rally. The HSK rally cost the city an astounding $650,000. There were only nine members who came, and they stood behind a fence that was bordered by a wall of police officers. The Klan was vastly outnumbered by people who had gathered to counterprotest their rally.

Tensions were running extremely high, as the HSK group were open carrying weapons, as were others in the counterprotest crowd. Antifa members were there as well, and you could feel the thick hostility in the air. I knew that all it would take was for one person to do something stupid and we would have a riot on our hands.

When the HSK leader started to yell into his little megaphone, his voice was drowned out by the chants of the citizens who gathered at the rally. They yelled things such as "No hatin' in Dayton!" A church group sang

"Amazing Grace" over a speaker, and people held signs and flags denouncing hate. I was on edge the entire time, waiting for someone to make a wrong move.

Thankfully, it was a peaceful rally. The hate group stormed our city with messages of hate and division, only to be met with peaceful citizens standing in solidarity against them. All differences were set aside and we thought we were in the clear from danger. It felt like a big win for our small town. However, we had no idea what was coming. Just two days later, we were pummeled with catastrophic tornados.

I was driving the engine at Station 15's, and we knew a big storm was moving in. Without knowing anything scientific about weather, you could just walk outside and be able to tell that a significant storm was rolling in. Having experienced bad storms on shift, I told my crew that I was going to take a nap, because it would probably be a long night of calls. I took a nap and woke up to tones that a tornado had hit and collapsed a house with people trapped inside of it, about fifteen minutes from our station. That was a pretty long haul, especially in an emergency situation. We raced down the highway and then turned onto Route 4, and when we turned the corner, everything was pitch black except for Children's Hospital, which was on a back-up generator. The entire power grid had been knocked out. It was eerie driving in complete darkness.

We quickly realized that there were tornados coming down all over the place. Someone on the engine said that there was a tornado touching down in Beavercreek, where I live, and I was freaking out not knowing if Lauren and the kids were okay. Driving the engine, I couldn't even check on them right away to make sure they were okay. We got off the highway and there were so many downed trees blocking the road, we couldn't even get to the house to which we'd been dispatched. Thankfully another crew was able to get there and help the people trapped inside the house. It was incredibly stressful trying to navigate the engine through the debris that were all over the place.

As I had predicted earlier, we were up all night going on runs. We were continuously being dispatched over wires that had fallen, checking buildings for fires as well as making sure people were able to evacuate from collapsed buildings. We were still out responding to calls when the sun finally came up in the morning. It was then we saw the devastating damage from the tornados. Roofs of houses and buildings were peeled off, bricks and shingles in heaps all over the place. Entire homes and buildings had collapsed, leaving a few lone walls standing. Cars had been lifted off the ground and thrown like tiny toys. Giant trees were completely uprooted and tossed all over the place. Hundreds of wires were down, dangerously hanging or fallen on the streets. I was astonished that an act of nature could cause so much damage. I'd never seen anything quite like this in my life. The damage was erratic, as one house would be untouched, and the house right beside it would be collapsed and reduced to rubble.

There were fifteen tornados that touched down in Dayton that night. One was a confirmed level EF4 tornado, with winds measuring up to 170 miles an hour. There ended up being a billion dollars' worth of damage in our city. It would take years to rebuild everything that was ruined. Our city had just peacefully made it through a hate rally, only to become obliterated by fifteen tornados. The saving grace was that, as a city, we'd just become a united front. We'd need the strength and help of everyone to get the city back on its' feet. We remained resilient, even after the devastating blows we received. We had no way of knowing that things were about to get much worse than any of us ever could've imagined. In three short months, our entire city would be rocked, and we would grieve and unite on a whole new level.

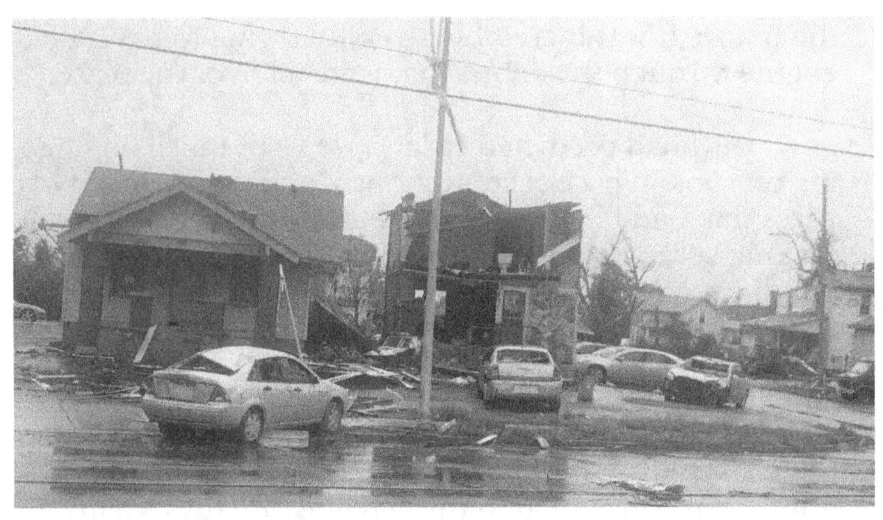

The twister aftermath

25 – OREGON DISTRICT

"Some stories won't have a happy ending, but there's always hope that the next one will. Hope is everything. Even when there's nothing else. Especially when there's nothing else."
-Clara Kensie - Aftermath

I woke up to a ton of missed calls and voicemails the morning of August 4th, 2019. My stomach dropped before I even listened to the voicemails, knowing that something was wrong. The magnitude of what happened was so much worse than I had anticipated. While I was safely tucked in my bed asleep, there had been a mass shooting.

The Oregon District is a gem within the city of Dayton. It's a historic area, with Federal and Queen Anne styled homes that were built in the 1800's. The streets are made of brick, giving the area a distinctive nostalgic feel. It's filled with art galleries, coffee shops, bars, pubs, restaurants, and a very popular comedy club. On the weekends the streets are closed so that people can safely walk around the area, giving it a miniature Bourbon Street feel. If you live in Dayton, chances are that you've most likely hung out in the Oregon District. It was a safe place to go have fun, so small if you didn't know about it you would miss it.

The Oregon District will no longer be known as the hidden gem in Dayton, but as the location of a deadly mass shooting. A man appeared with an AR loaded with a hundred-round drum magazine, and in cold blood started shooting. He just mowed people down. There were nine people who died in this shooting, including the shooter's sister. There were dozens of people who were shot or injured. As you can imagine, in the hysteria that ensued, people began running away from him, many into the doors of a nearby bar. The shooter was approaching the doors when Dayton Police shot and killed him before he could take any more lives. The police officers who responded to the scene were brave heroes. They stopped him thirty-two seconds after the first shot rang out.

Thirty-two seconds was all it took to shatter an entire city. The city was forever changed in less than one minute. The police cars and medics sped to the scene, anyone and everyone available to come was called upon. There was talk of a second shooter on the radios, and the district fire chief made the call for firefighters and medics to hang back. They were ordered not to enter the scene. If there was a second shooter, they didn't have a way to defend themselves. The police were overwhelmed with fatalities and injured people. They desperately needed the medics and firefighters to jump in and help. They had to load injured people into the backs of their cruisers and transport them to the hospital themselves. The firefighters and medics with adrenaline pumping though their veins were struggling to not break protocol and help. By the time it was confirmed that there wasn't a second shooter, the police had already tended to most of the injured people.

Animosity was born between the firefighters and police officers. The police called the firefighters "second responders", and the firefighters were angry they were being chastised for following their orders. In a lot of cities, there is tension between the police and firefighters, but in Dayton there was a strong comradery between the two. We were all on the same team and respected each other. That was just another thing that was shattered during this shooting.

That night, police and firefighters experienced an evil that was beyond comprehension. Firefighters that responded to the event were ordered to attend a mandatory debriefing, called critical incident stress debriefing (CISD). This debriefing did not go over well. The crews just wanted to go home and sleep. A lot of them were still processing what had happened, and it was too soon to force them to talk about the shooting. This would be the last time that the CISD model would be utilized in our city. Following this tragedy, the decision was made to follow the peer-support model in the future. This model did not require attendance of those involved in traumatic events and allowed crews to talk when they were ready.

The aftermath to a shooting like this was horrific. The shooting took place around one in the morning, so when the sun came up, firefighters were dispatched to clean the scene. Random shoes littered the streets, as people lost them literally running for their lives. Windows were peppered with bullet holes. I'm trying not to get too graphic, but there was blood everywhere. There was a nauseating stench from the spilled blood that hung in the air. The city leaders wanted to set up a stage near the scene, to rally the city together and honor those who had lost their lives. To get the scene stage- and camera-ready, the firefighters used their hoses to spray the blood away. Not all of it washed away from the pressure of the hose water. This forced crews on their hands and knees, scrubbing away bloodstains with tiny brushes. The stains might have lifted from the ground, but they forever stayed on those who responded to the shooting.

When the scene reopened to the public, makeshift shrines quickly appeared, honoring those who had lost their lives. The sidewalks were covered with beautiful flowers and candles. Tears spilled where blood had filled the streets. Fear loomed in the eyes of brokenhearted residents. The words "Dayton Strong" were found all over the city—chalkboard signs, store windows, and spraypainted on abandoned buildings. The people in Dayton were shattered, but they rallied as a community, understanding that the evil actions of one person didn't get to be the legacy that was left behind. White doves were released in honor of those who had lost their lives. The doves symbolize peace, and though we didn't feel it in the moment, we hoped that eventually peace would replace grief.

I felt really guilty I didn't hear my phone ring and join my brothers and sisters responding to the shooting. If I'm being honest, I also felt a sense of relief I wasn't one of the responders; the relief only fueled my guilt. I was slotted to be on the peer-support team for Dayton but hadn't undergone the training yet. If you are unfamiliar with the term, peer support is a team of firefighters that assist members who are struggling to cope with trauma. They can develop and vet resources that fellow firefighters can trust. The vital key to this group is that they understand and can relate to the nature of the job, unlike others who are not involved in the fire service. The IAFF Disaster Team and State Peer Teams were called. I accompanied them to the various stations, checking on members. This was the same approach I would later take in another tragedy, but it would land me in trouble.

There were therapy dogs that came with us to the stations, and it was the first time I had ever really experienced the benefits of these animals firsthand. Their presence helped calm anxious members and eased some of them into opening up about how they were really doing. Years later, I would revisit the idea of therapy dogs and pursue getting one to benefit the members in our city.

I spoke to Jeff Orrange, who was a part of the peer-support team in Orlando. I talked to him about how a lot of our members were really struggling with the way that everything happened. Following direct orders, they'd been unable to utilize their thorough training and help in a crisis. He told me that there's a term for how they were feeling called 'moral injury.' This term was derived from the military, and it describes having to do something that goes against your morals. They wanted to jump in and help more than anything; being told to hang back went against every fiber of their being. The symptoms to this are very similar to the symptoms of post-traumatic stress disorder (PTSD).

The IAFF suggested we gather all of the first responders at an event where they could experience some normalcy and unwind with people who understood what they were going through. I helped organize "First Responder Night." This took place at the Dublin Pub, a restaurant that directly faces the Oregon District (where the shooting took place). The event helped mend the fractured trust between the police and firefighters. We granted each other permission to simply 'not be okay.' It was a baby step in the right direction towards healing.

Years later when I was in my role on the peer-support team and wellness coordinator, I talked with a lot of people that were still struggling from the trauma of this event.

Comedian Dave Chapelle, who lives in a suburb of Dayton, organized an incredible benefit concert called the Gem City Shine to honor the victims of the shooting. He arranged for several comedians and musicians to perform, topping the night off with Stevie Wonder as the show's headliner. Jon Stewart was also there, and I had the opportunity to personally thank him for all of the advocacy he has done on behalf of firefighters. This benefit helped the citizens of Dayton reclaim their beloved city out of the hands of evil.

After the shooting occurred, President Trump also came to Dayton to pay his respects. I had the privilege of being chosen to be a part of his motorcade. I had a secret service agent riding in the medic with me, which was a pretty surreal experience. He gave me a button to wear to show I had been vetted and approved, and the button basically kept me from getting shot by his security team. Trump flew Air Force One into Wright Patterson Air Force Base, and I was one of the many vehicles in the motorcade escorting him from there to the Oregon District, as well as Miami Valley Hospital. Trump met with the police officers who took the shooter down, as well as some of the leaders in the fire department. Regardless of where you stand politically, it was a once-in-a-lifetime experience for me, and I was excited to have a small part in Trump's visit.

People will sometimes say things like, "It takes a special person to do the job you do." While that statement is true, it doesn't negate the fact that although we choose to run into dangerous situations, we aren't immune to grief and trauma. It doesn't matter how tough or brave one thinks they are; no human is a match for looking this kind of evil in the eye.

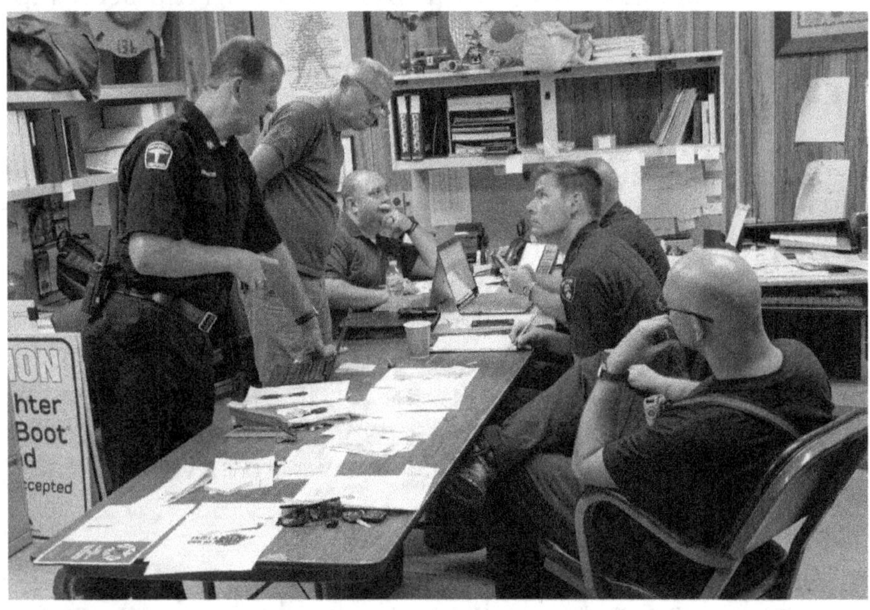

The department and union on a conference call with leaders from the IAFF following the Oregon District mass shooting

26 – THE 25 LIVE

"The hardest thing to do is to be true to yourself, especially when everybody is watching."
-Dave Chapelle

I had experienced an insurmountable amount of grief and trauma within the past few months, and one place I turned to for solace was James Geering's podcast, "Behind the Shield." It's a large-scale health and wellness podcast, where James interviews men and women who serve our communities (firefighters, police officers, military members) and gleans wellness tips and advice applicable to first responders. There weren't a lot of these types of podcasts, and I felt inspired to start my own.

I started "The 25 Live," my own version of a health and wellness podcast. The number twenty-five is significant for a lot of firefighters, because we typically have to work for twenty-five years before we can retire. I had created a list of twenty-five things to do to prevent getting occupational cancer. It was only fitting that I name my podcast "The 25 Live." The idea is to take all of the precautions possible in order to stay healthy and alive on the job, and be able to enjoy retirement after putting in twenty-five years of work.

My initial goal was to record one podcast a week. I had a variety of guests come on and share their wealth of knowledge on a particular topic. I didn't realize it until recently, but looking back through my podcast, I can see that it's a direct reflection of whatever I was going through at that moment in time. I had experts come on and talk about topics I was struggling through, and I didn't see this trend until I looked back at the queue of the episodes.

I loved hosting the podcast. I was learning a lot of valuable information from successful people that were very insightful and experienced. It took a lot of time planning and preparing for the episodes. For example, if I was interviewing someone who just came out with a book, I wanted to make sure I read their book so that I could ask them relevant questions and help promote it. I felt as though it was the respect I owed my guests for taking the time to talk with me.

After about a year of cranking out weekly podcasts, I was brought onto the "Fire Engineering" podcast, doing one podcast a month for them. I was excited to get this opportunity, as they have already curated an established audience of dedicated listeners. It was difficult keeping up with five podcasts a month, but I maintained it up until I received my cancer diagnosis. Everything changed when I learned I had cancer.

My podcasts went from interviewing guests to essentially being a real-time vocal diary where I talked about what was happening in my cancer journey. I did this for a couple of reasons. One, it was super cathartic to vocalize how I was feeling. I allowed myself to be raw and vulnerable in these episodes. I just let myself feel whatever emotion I was feeling at the time. Sometimes I was grateful that it wasn't a worse circumstance, and sometimes I was angry I was even dealing with cancer. Sometimes I was really anxious and fearful of what was to come. I took everyone along with me on the ups and downs of my journey. Another reason I chose to stop the format I had been doing with interviewing guests was because it was easier to give one update than make thirty different phone calls. It was a really emotional time for me, and that's obvious if you listen to those particular episodes. I even had Lauren come on for an episode and talk about my cancer journey from her perspective.

I'm in a much different place right now than I was when I first started my podcast. I only record one a month, and that is the show I contribute to the "Fire Engineering" podcast. With everything I've gone through, my priorities have shifted, and that was one thing I had to take off of my plate.

Recently I have been interviewed on other podcasts, and it's cool being on the other side of things. I was pretty excited when "the podfather" himself, James Geering, invited me to come on his show as a guest. It was a full-circle moment for me, as his podcast is what had inspired me to begin my own. Like everything else in my life, this wasn't ever part of my plan; but I think it's way better.

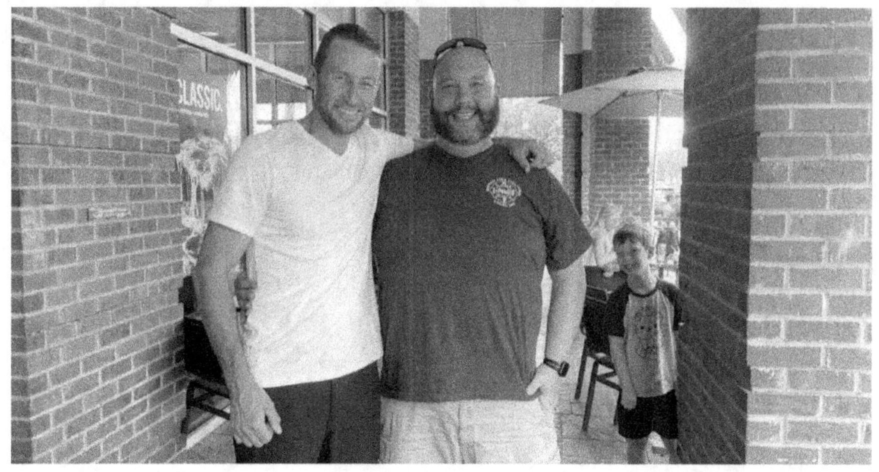

James Geering & I in Ocala (photobomb by Jameson)

27 – TAHOE

I was enjoying running my cancer-consulting company. Through my podcast and business, I felt like the awareness I was bringing to various firehouses was opening their eyes to the dangers that lurked among them, forcing them to make changes. When I landed a consulting gig with the fire department in South Lake Tahoe, I was pumped. It isn't every day you get the opportunity to work in a beautiful area such as South Lake Tahoe. I brought Lauren with me, excited to explore the exquisite area together when I wasn't working. We arrived and I got right to work. The consulting work at the station in South Lake Tahoe was going well, and in between classes I would get a coffee and relax on a bench by the lake. It was October, and I was surrounded by trees donning the bright red, orange, and yellow colors of sunset. I felt energized by the serenity of the area.

I had a day off from teaching classes, so Lauren and I were excited to explore Lake Tahoe together. We were waiting to be seated at a restaurant when I received a text saying that a friend and fellow firefighter had died by suicide. They called our name to seat us, and frozen in disbelief, I stumbled over to the table. The news slowly started to sink in, and the highly recommended restaurant no longer mattered. We excused ourselves and went to a picnic table on the beach next to the restaurant. I felt an overwhelming sense of helplessness. My crew were the ones to go on-scene and find our coworker, our brother, dead. I needed to make sure they were okay—surely, they were not. How could this have happened? As the initial shock wore off, I felt overwhelmed with sadness over the loss of a great friend. I was the one who typically headed up funeral arrangements, but I couldn't do any of that from across the country.

I reached out to my friend Jeff Orrange to try and figure out how to navigate this situation. Jeff asked the simple question, "Does South Lake Tahoe have a peer-support team?" I didn't know the answer, so I gave Mike a call. Mike helped connect me to Leslie, who was his captain and a peer supporter. Leslie and her group rallied around me, and I stayed and finished out my commitment to teach the last day of classes.

During that last day, I took a break and wandered over to the bench I had sat at the past few days, and something immediately caught my eye. On the bench was a small wooden cross from a rosary. In general, I tried to avoid religion and spirituality, but even I couldn't deny the significance of the cross. In the middle of His breathtaking creation, I felt God meeting me in the midst of my pain. I knew that there was a plan much bigger than what my mind could comprehend. I had a lot of uncertainty, but in that moment, I knew that God had a plan, I was a part of it, and He was at work. I took the cross home with me, along with a newfound hope in God.

Down the line, I was asked to go back to Tahoe for more consulting work, but I declined the offer. Tahoe in all of its beauty had become tainted by the fear and helplessness I'd experienced while visiting; I couldn't bear facing it again. A few years later, another offer was made for a friend and I to go out there, and I knew it was time to face my fears. We went to Tahoe and found ourselves on the very bench on which I'd found the cross. Along with a small piece of me, I left the wooden cross on the bench, knowing that someone else would need the hope it gave me.

Although I didn't know it at the time, the death of my friend heavily impacted me, and would later become a catalyst for change in our policies at the station.

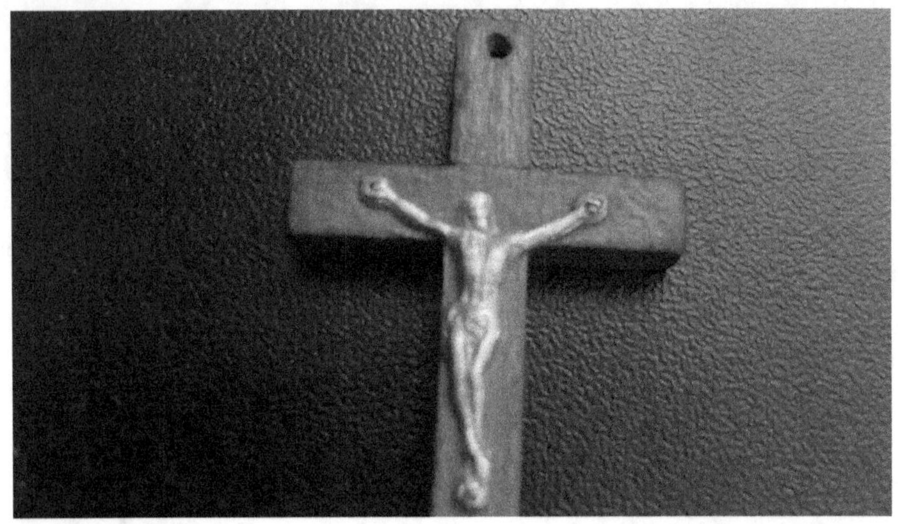

The rosary cross I found on the bench in South Lake Tahoe

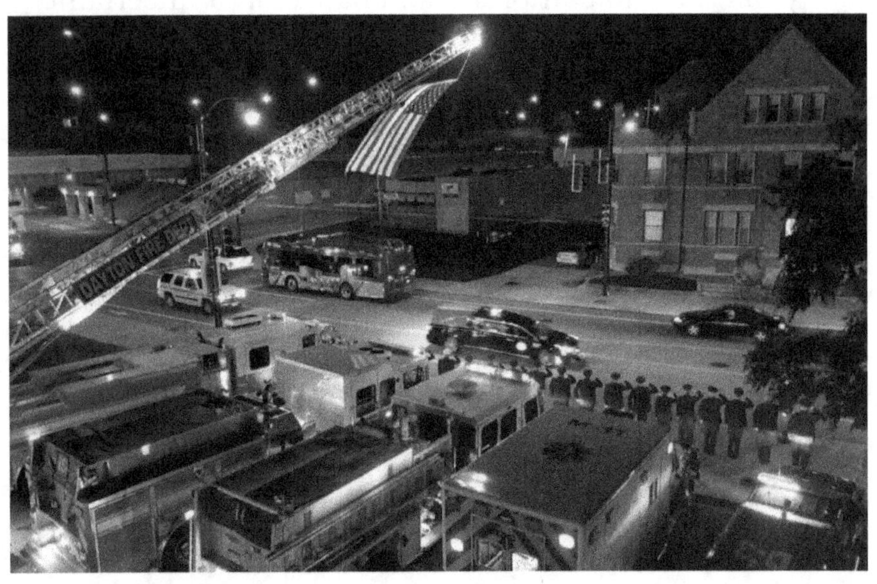

Brian's funeral procession passing Station 11

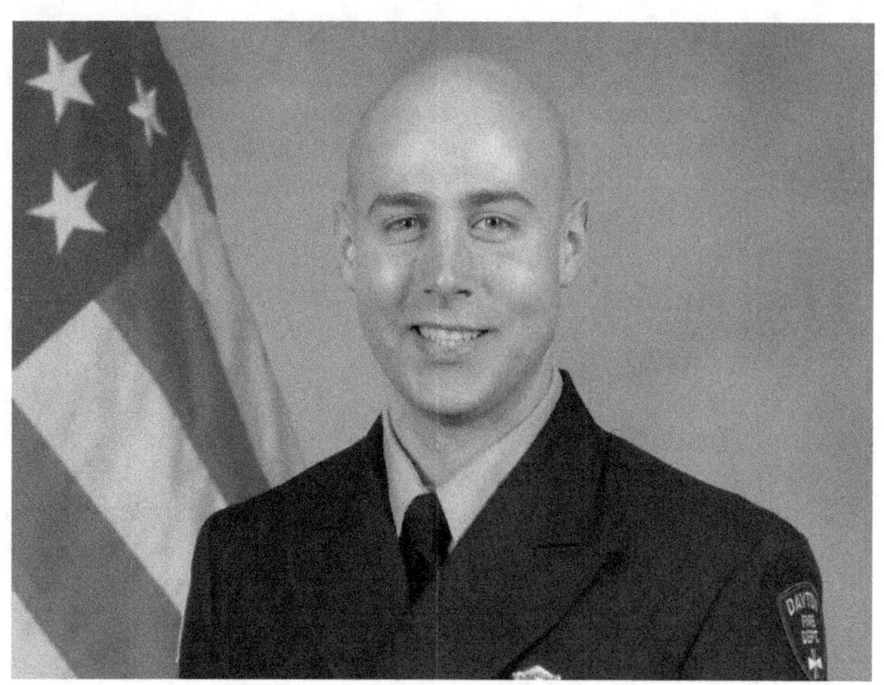

Briane Poole
11/2/1983 – 10/9/2019

"When it comes to life, the critical thing is whether you take things for granted or take them with gratitude."
-Gilbert K. Chesterton

I almost didn't include this chapter, because like everyone else, I'm sick and tired of hearing about Covid. However, the virus changed everything, especially my job. It would be remiss of me to leave it out. In March of 2020 when Covid became official, I was on vacation. The whole plan was for everything to shut down for just two weeks to flatten the curve. I was super annoyed with this, mainly because they canceled the NCAA tournament, and the University of Dayton's basketball team was ranked third. The cancellation of the basketball tournament would quickly become the least of my concerns.

I was relieved I was on vacation when they decided to close everything for two weeks. The curve would flatten just in time for me to return from vacation. We all know how that went. Two weeks stretched into two months, and we wouldn't return to a feeling of normalcy for years.

Covid affected everything about my job. The personal protective equipment (PPE) that we had to wear for every run was extremely uncomfortable, not to mention added time for us to get on scene. When we had to go into a nursing home, it felt like we were entering an alternate reality. We had to unzip huge plastic curtains to get into the facility, and then again to gain access to the rooms. The masks were uncomfortable, and we couldn't smile at any of the patients, taking away a simple means of comforting them. Over the course of the past few years, we have picked up a ton of patients who were really sick with Covid and transported them to the hospital.

Lauren is a nurse, and both of our jobs were considered essential. Neither of us were able to work from home during this daunting time. This made it difficult when the school shut down and shifted to remote learning. Luckily my parents were able to jump in and help with our boys.

We ended up getting sick with Covid on Thanksgiving. I love getting together with my family and eating really good food, but that year we were isolated at our house. My parents dropped food off on our porch for us, and while I appreciated the gesture, I couldn't taste one bite of anything I ate. I longed to be at my parents' house with the rest of the family, indulging in turkey and mashed potatoes. In the grand scheme of things, it sounds super petty to be complaining about missing a holiday meal and get-together. The virus took things away, both on a small and large scale. We experienced loss on both ends of the spectrum. Thankfully, nobody in my family had any life-altering complications after being sick. A friend of mine, Jeff, a firefighter in Washington Township, passed away from complications after having Covid. I did peer support at his station in Washington Township, the station where I started out working as a firefighter.

The culture at the station drastically changed. Per regulations, we were no longer allowed to congregate together between runs. We separated throughout the station so that we didn't have to wear a mask twenty-four hours a day. It was extremely isolating, taking away the comradery we were accustomed to having at work. It was common to be at work one day, and then someone that was on shift with you call the following day to apologize, saying that they had just tested positive for Covid. I'd say it was a roller coaster, but there weren't really any positive things coming out of the virus. It was a long, downhill slide, gaining momentum the longer this went on.

I know that it wasn't just my profession that experienced negative impacts to our mental health, but society in general. We were not created to be isolated from each other, but in community with one another. The only good thing that has come out of Covid, is that I'll never take little things for granted as I had before the epidemic. The whole world had the rug pulled out from under us. Sadly, not everyone was able to stand back up again. I'm thankful just to be alive. There are so many things I'll never take for granted again the way I did in the past. Some of these include my fire family eating meals together, hanging out between calls, and not having to bunk in separate parts of the station. The nature of our job bonds us, because a lot of people don't understand what we go through on a daily basis. Taking away that comradery had such a negative impact on all of us. It was awful going on hard runs, and then coming back to the station and being isolated from everyone.

I also came to appreciate a multitude of things in my personal life, such as the kids actually attending school versus remote learning, getting to play sports again, going out to eat at restaurants, and concerts and shows coming back. The list goes on and on.

I would venture to say that none of us are the same as before the Covid epidemic rocked our world; perhaps we are all a little better. We understand how the world can change on a dime and saw firsthand that tomorrow isn't guaranteed. We love a little harder, take more risks, and value simple pleasures that were taken from us. Covid took a lot away, but also gave us new perspective and appreciation for life.

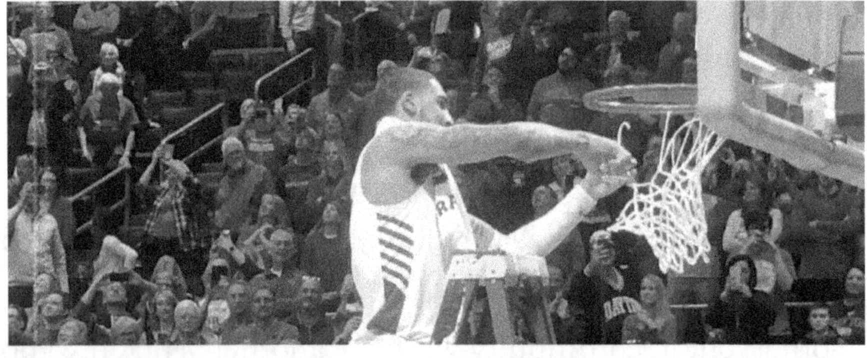

What could have been. Thanks a lot Covid!

29 – ROCKIN' ROD

"It's funny to think about the things in your life that can make you cry just knowing that they existed, can then become the same thing that make you cry knowing that they're now gone. I think those things come into our lives to help us get from one place to a better one."
-Ted Lasso

Gaining perspective for how precious life is leads me to sharing about one of the greatest men I've ever met, Rod Longpre'. My first interaction with Rod Longpre' was January 29th, 2001 at 0700 in the morning. It was my first day at Dayton Fire Drill School. I sat in the front row, and at 0700 the tones went off and Rod kicked in the door and yelled at us to get on our feet. He continued to berate us as if we were in the opening scene of *Full Metal Jacket.* He scared the crap out of me.

I remember being at home later that night thinking, "What did I just get myself into?" I was a punk twenty-one-year-old, and things just got real, fast. There were two double classes of twenty, so my class had to move away from the training center. This meant I didn't have to deal with Drill Sergeant Rod. We came back to do a mass casualty drill, and as soon as I saw Rod I thought, "Here we go again." He got on the bus and screamed at us to get off his bus, so we scrambled off as fast as we could.

When we finished EMT training, Rod was the one who led us in our physical training (PT). He dropped the drill sergeant act, and we got to know the real Rod; Rockin' Rod. He gained our respect, (not just because we were afraid of him) but because he was the real deal. He was not only a rockstar firefighter, but a musical rockstar as well. Rod was super talented and could play several instruments. He volunteered to play at the Team Gavin benefit we threw, and everyone loved his music. Having served in the army, he was big into the Honor Guard.

The week I graduated, the instructors were telling us where we'd been assigned. I still remember them announcing, "Burneka, 15-3."

Rod, who worked at that station, pointed at me and said, "Your ass belongs to me."

During the few years I got to work with Rod, he was a mentor in the firehouse, but also beyond that. He understood that being a firefighter was a calling and did his best to show me the ropes. He also didn't shy away from hard conversations. Even when it was extremely taboo to talk about feelings, Rod would express the post-traumatic stress he was experiencing. He cracked a door that not many would walk through, let alone open, especially during that time period. Rod and I were bunkmates when we were at 15's. Every night as we would touch our heads to our pillows, he would say, "Jim, tell me a story," in an innocent, childlike manner. It always made me laugh. I do that same voice to my boys sometimes.

Rod's favorite story to share about me came from an unfortunate laundry accident that he witnessed. I'd just come back from a call in which I ended up with blood on my uniform. I changed clothes and decided to wash my soiled uniform in the station's clothes washer and dryer. My friend Tim was kind enough to let me use his liquid fabric softener. This liquid fabric softener was foreign to me. I was used to the dryer-sheet fabric softeners. I knew that the dryer sheets went into the dryer, so I assumed that the liquid fabric softener would as well. Imagine Rod watching TV in the apparatus bay, and in the corner of his eye he sees me throwing liquid fabric softener into the dryer. I'll never forget his inquisitive statement, "Jim, what are you doing?" An important lesson was learned that day, and I haven't made that mistake ever again.

Rod was one of the creators of the Miami Valley Firefighter/EMS Memorial. He had procured some land where the memorial would eventually be built. I was honored to help him fundraise over $100,000 to have the memorial commissioned. It was a beautiful space, and we would hold our annual memorial services there.

Rod and I remained close while we worked at different stations, as well as after he retired. He had become an irreplaceable part of my support system. When Lauren and I were planning our wedding, I threw out his name to be the officiant. Lauren agreed that Rod would be perfect for the job. He became an ordained minister, just so that he could officiate our wedding. He did an amazing job, and it was such an honor for him to play such an important role at our wedding. I'm forever grateful that our cherished wedding photos include my mentor and friend, Rod.

A few years later, Rod was diagnosed with liver cancer. He stayed very active throughout his battle with cancer, and he beat it. Everyone was so relieved he had dodged that bullet.

Unbeknownst to us, a few years after he beat cancer, he was diagnosed with it again. This time, it was throughout his stomach. He didn't tell us until the very end when he was in hospice care. I'm one of the few people who was able to talk to him while he was still coherent. I'd arranged to get a hospital bed to his house to keep him comfortable. He would only use it for one afternoon.

I told him I loved him, and he said it back to me. Despite the dire circumstances, he had a calmness and peace about him. A lot of people were coming to see Rod, and I had to get to my son's practice. I left and drove to the Kettering YMCA. As I pulled into the parking lot, I got a call that Rod had left the earth. Only twenty minutes had passed since I was with him. I couldn't believe in this short amount of time he had died.

I left the parking lot and drove back to Rod's house, where we called our medics to come to the scene so they could take him to the funeral home. I don't know if it was the best decision, but I chose to ride in the back of the medic with him. I was trying to do right by him, but it was one of the most difficult things I have done. I know it is uncustomary to be in such close proximity to a loved one's deceased body. But Rod had looked after me since I was a rookie, shepherding me along the way throughout my career and life outside of my career. The least I could do was look after his body and ensure he got to the funeral home.

I'd just lost one of the most influential and precious people in my life, yet I didn't allow myself the time or space to grieve. I did what I'd always done and jumped full steam ahead into planning mode. Rod lived an extraordinary life. He left everything and everyone better than he found them. He was the best at giving tough love as well as encouragement. He could always distinguish which one you needed. Rod was selfless and beloved by everyone. Not just our Dayton members, but people from all over loved and respected Rod.

Planning his service was a little tricky, because it was in October of 2020, so Covid was an issue. We couldn't hold a ceremony indoors with all of the restrictions put in place. I brought up the idea of having his funeral at the Miami Valley Firefighter/EMS Memorial, and miraculously, it was approved. It wasn't a holy place, but it was sacred to us. We wanted to give Rod the best going-away party there ever was.

The day of his funeral, the on-duty members solemnly stood outside of their stations as the funeral procession passed, paying tribute to Rod and his family. Nick Mitchell played "The Star-Spangled Banner" on an electric guitar, the chords reverberating across the fall-colored leaves. There was a twenty-one-gun salute honoring his days in the army, the echo of the shots exploding across the sky. Bagpipers played long, drawn-out notes that seemed to float off into Heaven. Though his loss was devastating, we celebrated the way that he lived.

Rod had known that his death was imminent. He took the time, which he didn't have a lot of left, to pen a goodbye note. The note was Rod's creed, how he lived his life, and his encouragement for others to do the same. See for yourself:

"So live your life that the fear of death can never enter your heart. Trouble no one about their religion, respect others in their view and demand that they respect yours. Love your life, perfect your life, beautify all things in your life. Seek to make your life long and its purpose the service of the people. Prepare a noble death song for the day when you go over the great divide. Always give a word or sign of salute when meeting a passing friend. Show respect to all people and grovel to none. When you arise in the morning, give thanks for the food and for the joy of living. If you see no reason for giving thanks, then the fault lies only in yourself. Abuse no one and no thing, for abuse turns wise ones to fools and robs the spirit of its vision. When it comes your time to die, be not like those whose hearts are filled with the fear of death, so that when their time comes, they weep and pray for a little more time to live their lives over again in a different way. Sing your death song like a hero going home."

-Rod Longpre' (Sings with Eagles)

After the funeral was over, I melted behind the memorial and finally grieved over the deep loss of my friend. I am talking snotty, red-faced, barely breathing, ugly cried. Rod had put his blood, sweat, and tears into this memorial, and now some of his ashes would lie here too.

It always bothered me and some of Rod's friends that we were never able to give Rod an appropriate send-off due to Covid. When Covid restrictions finally calmed down in 2022, some of Rod's friends and I put together a musical celebration in remembrance of him. We had a great evening with lots of Rod's friends and raised several thousand dollars for upkeep of the Miami Valley

Firefighter/EMS Memorial that he'd worked so hard at creating.

I was supposed to go to Colorado Springs where Rod would be honored at the IAFF Fallen Firefighter Memorial. Instead, I landed in Maryland, at the Center of Excellence. I had a lot of inner turmoil over this decision. I even had an internal dialogue with Rod about the situation. I felt like I owed it to him to honor his life and legacy in Colorado Springs. I could hear him telling me that I owed it to myself to get healthy again. He made such an impact on me, that even after he left the earth, I knew exactly how he would guide me.

Perhaps the best way to honor him was not to witness his name on the memorial, but to ensure that my name would not be added to it as well.

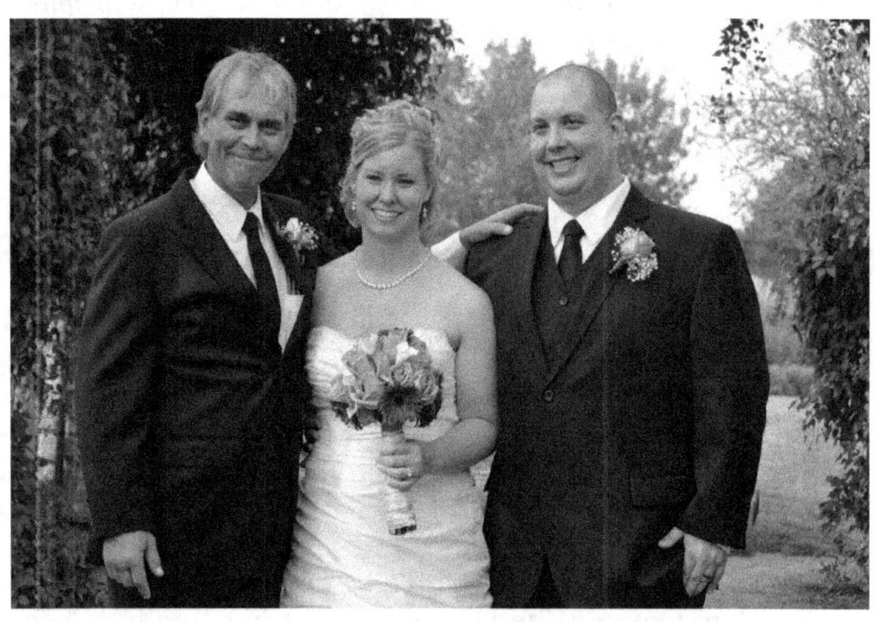

Rod, Lauren and me on our wedding day

30 – CANCER

"The best view comes after the hardest climb."
- Benjamin Franklin

My heart was not in good shape after losing Rod, and I'd soon find out that my body was not well either. Mark Rhine is a friend of mine who opened my eyes to the reality of cancer. His wife found a spot on his lower back that she wanted him to get looked at. He put it off for quite some time, being a busy father to five children and working. When he finally went to the doctor to get the spot looked at, he learned that he had terminal cancer—stage 4 melanoma. Following his diagnosis, Mark would come and talk to our rookies about the importance of early detection.

This story stayed in the back of my mind, so when Lauren told me she thought the right side of my neck looked bigger than the left, I made an appointment to get it looked at. I was fairly confident everything would check out fine, as I couldn't see a difference when I looked in the mirror and I didn't have any symptoms.

I went to the doctor's office and they found a small nodule that he said we would monitor, and they casually told me to come back in a year or two for another scan. I made an appointment for the following year, confident that everything was fine, but erring on the side of caution.

The next year I returned for my scheduled appointment to do another scan of the nodule. As I was leaving the office, I got a notification that the nodule had grown. I had an appointment to get a biopsy done the next day.

Lauren and I went to a pathologist, and I had the biopsy taken. The doctor excused himself from the room with the biopsy to examine it. He came back less than ten minutes later with a small note that read, "Papillary thyroid carcinoma. Most common type of thyroid cancer. Least aggressive. Requires surgery."

I had been doing my job of consulting with departments trying to reduce the risk of obtaining occupational cancer for quite some time now. I felt as though I was well-versed in this area and understand the risks associated with my profession. But nothing can prepare you for a cancer diagnosis. I felt numb as we left the office. On the way home I called my Bureau of Workers Compensation attorney, knowing this is the first call I advise members to make after receiving a diagnosis. As the numbness wore off and reality sank in, I felt very anxious, scared, and hypocritical. I was the guy who traveled around trying to reduce the risk of occupational cancer, but here I was, being diagnosed myself. Who was going to take me seriously after this? How would I explain it to my kids, who were only four and seven years old? A million questions began to run through my mind.

Lauren carried a lot of the weight throughout this entire process. She exemplified strength and grace. I knew it wasn't fair, but I asked her to tell my family and close friends that I had cancer. I struggled to even get the words out of my mouth, let alone watch them dissolve into sadness over the news. She also was the one who asked the hard questions at the doctor's office, taking notes and then explaining to me later once I came out of my fog. Do you remember watching *Charlie Brown* when you were a kid? You could hear his teacher talking but couldn't understand what she was saying. That's exactly how I felt at the doctor's appointments; I could hear them talking, but I wasn't processing anything they were saying. I have to credit Lauren for taking charge and doing what I couldn't at the time.

Both our families were extremely supportive while we were going through this. I knew that if we needed anything at all, all I had to do was pick up the phone and ask.

A lot of people were praying for me, and it was really comforting to know I had such a strong support system.

As mentioned previously in this book, I had a falling-out with the FCSN. I knew it might not be well received, but I reached out to them asking for support. The president of the organization put our grievances aside, and the support they offered me was incredible. They sent me a toolbox that was prominent in dealing with doctor's appointments and talking to my children about cancer. I hate that it took a cancer diagnosis for me to fix that relationship, but I'm thankful that we have come full circle, as I am currently a mentor for their organization.

There were several places where I could go to have the surgery to remove my cancer. We chose to proceed with the Ohio State James Cancer Center. I had to wait about a month to have the surgery. I know a month isn't long, but it felt as though years had passed during that time. Knowing that something that could kill me was in my body made me incredibly anxious. I wanted it out the moment I knew it was in there. When I got there and was waiting in the pre-op holding area, there was a patient across from me who looked really sick. She was extremely thin, bald, and weak. It snapped me out of feeling sorry for myself and put into perspective that while any cancer is serious, my situation could be so much worse than it was.

I had surgery, and they removed the isthmus portion of my thyroid, getting the cancer out of my body. During the surgery, my oxygen levels dropped, so they kept me overnight to monitor me, which wasn't part of the original plan. That night I remember having the best Jell-O I've ever eaten in my life; I guess anything is amazing when you haven't eaten in over a day. I was doing better throughout the night, so they were able to remove the nasal cannula and additional equipment I was hooked up to. My hospital room overlooked the Ohio State football stadium. I remember dozing off and on while staring at "the Shoe."

During my recovery, I traveled to Sedona, Arizona, a place known for its unique red rocks, an environment where one could attain peace. While in Sedona, my doctor called me and said that the pathology report showed that cancer was found in my lymph nodes. The lymph nodes are commonly known as the highway to the body. The doctor was confident that the cancer had not spread anywhere else, and that he'd successfully removed it all, but it still sent me down a rabbit hole. I went from a relaxing, healing journey among the serene red rocks of Sedona to a very unhealthy mental state. Anxiety was zipping throughout my body. My depression began to spiral out of control. I couldn't shake the fear that cancer was unknowingly looming inside me.

I was off work for a few months recovering from surgery, and I asked my fire chief if there was a forty-hour a week position I could possibly work. It felt insane to me to go back into the very environment that I believe made me sick. Initially there wasn't a forty-hour position available, so I had to go back to work at the firehouse.

I had overcome my illness but didn't know how I'd be able to conquer the anxiety of my cancer coming back. Sometimes I wonder if the *fear* of the disease is worse than the disease itself. The poisonous cancer cells were removed from my body, yet fear still pulsed throughout my veins. I realized that healing my body was one thing; healing my mind was a much bigger feat than I could have imagined.

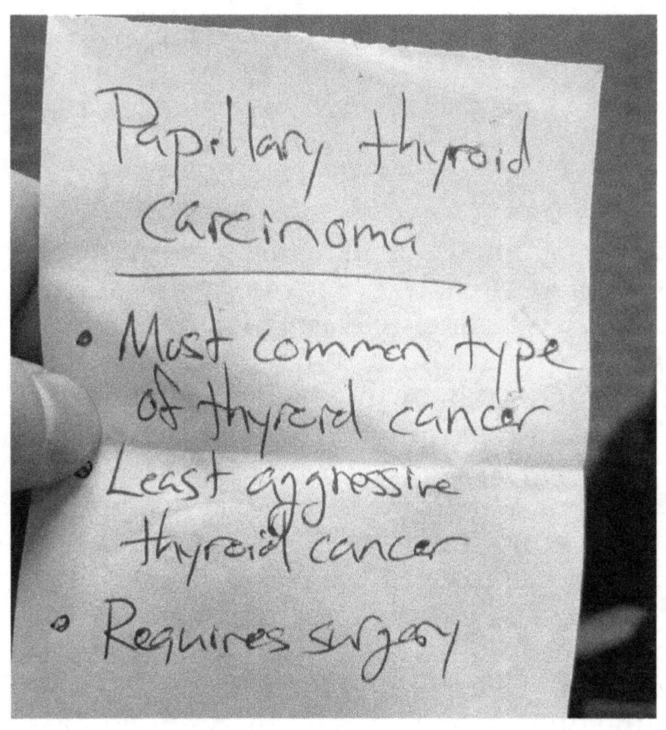

The note handed to me after my biopsy review

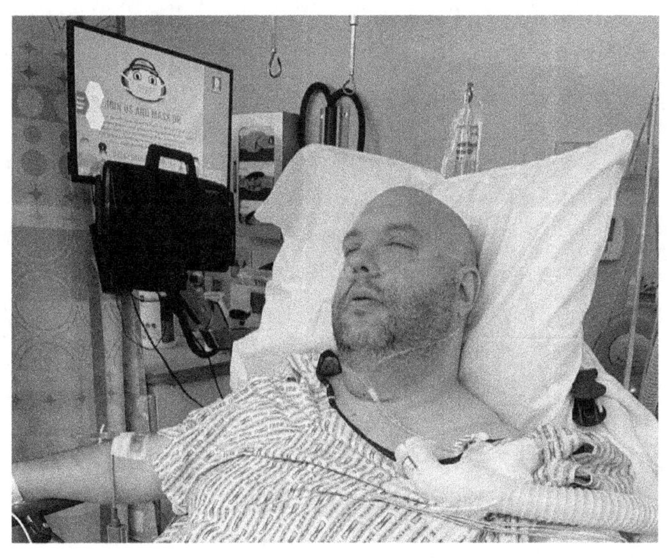

In the recovery room after surgery

31 – HONORING THE FALLEN

*"Oh yes, the past can hurt. But you can either run from it, or
learn from it"*
-Rafiki (The Lion King)

My mind was still reeling from the cancer I just had
removed from my body. It was truly divine intervention discovering I had cancer, as I didn't have
any symptoms and even my doctors weren't concerned. I
didn't understand why I had survived the disease, while
close friends of mine were not so lucky.

For quite some time, I had been brainstorming how
I could honor my friends who died in the line of duty. I finally landed on getting a tattoo. It wouldn't be a coy tattoo
that only I would know the meaning, I wanted to get
something that was an obvious tribute to friends of mine
who were fallen firefighters. I definitely went through a
tattoo phase when I was in my twenties. I wish I could tell
you that each one represents something deep and meaningful, but the truth is I just liked the way they looked. After I got that out of my system, I knew that if I were to get
any more tattoos, they would have to be meaningful to
me. I could not think of a more meaningful tattoo than
this.

I had a friend who'd recently gotten a tattoo in Columbus, and I was impressed with the way it had turned
out. He put me in touch with the artist he used, and I explained to her what I was wanting to do. I sent her some
photos of the IAFF Memorial with the logo, as well as the
names of my friends. She told me she would come up with
something along the lines of what I was thinking. I know
this sounds crazy, but I didn't see her finished design until
the morning I was getting the tattoo at her studio.

I was recovering from my cancer removal surgery,
so it was the optimal time to get a tattoo done. I was already restricted in what I could do and was off work. Some

people would say this tattoo was a result of survivor's guilt, a notion that I shoot down to this day. I had wanted to find a unique way to honor my friends and felt strongly this would be perfect.

When the tattoo artist showed me her design, I loved it. She incorporated every aspect that I wanted included in my tattoo. It was even better than I'd expected. I had her do the tattoo on the front of my right leg. Out of all of my tattoos, it hurt the most. The pain was a small price to pay for the daily reminder I have to live my life to the fullest, as well as remembering the sacrifice each name on my leg made.

There are seven names on my leg. I would like to tell you a little about each man:

Rod Longpre' - Rod is my Jedi Master Force ghost. All of my fellow nerds will understand what this means! The chapter "Rockin' Rod" elaborates on his life.

Bobby Hetzer - Bobby was such an incredible man. The chapter "Bobby" elaborates on his life.

Brian Poole - I used to see Brian every morning when he was getting off shift. Brian was an incredible guy. He was super friendly and well-liked. Brian was a dedicated firefighter and paramedic, who unfortunately saw a lot of really ugly things. Brian ended up dying by suicide. His death shook the department, as he was such a cherished person. We all felt the pain of his sudden death. I talked about Brian in more detail in the "Lake Tahoe" chapter.

Kevin Quinn - Kevin served as a lieutenant for Dayton as well as a paramedic. Kevin was hilarious, beloved by everyone. He was the life of the party. I always think about how funny he was. He unexpectedly died of a heart attack at the dispatch center. I still remember my captain getting the call about his death, and the disbelief and grief on his

face as he heard the news. We couldn't believe that someone so full of life was taken so abruptly.

Rickie Halcomb - Rickie was simply an awesome guy. He
was the union president when I first started on the job. He
was such an incredible leader. Rickie was forced to retire
earlier than he wanted to due to contracting hepatitis
while working the scene of a bad car accident. He continued to stay involved in the union, acting as the Fourth District president for the union. He spent the last few years of
his life in Florida, enjoying the sunshine and warmth before hepatitis claimed his life.

Eric Sondeen - Eric was the Colorado FCSN coordinator.
Eric retired as a lieutenant paramedic in Littleton, Colorado, after working in the fire rescue service for twenty-
eight years. He was a man who encompassed the gentlest
spirit. He had a motorcycle with a sidecar and used to
drive cancer patients around in the sidecar. Those patients
lost their ability to do many everyday tasks, so he gave
them the gift of freedom that only flying through the
open fresh air can give. He was so selfless and genuinely
had a heart for serving others.

Josh Comeau - Josh was a firefighter in South Bend, Indiana. Josh had the most infectious joy, and the moment I
met him, I knew that we would become close friends. I was
both in awe and astonished by the way that he lived his life
so full of love and joy. One day Josh passed out while driving the engine, wrecking into a car. It turned out that he
had a brain tumor. He had surgery on it and eventually returned to work. I was hired to do cancer consulting work
in South Bend, and Josh accompanied me to every training. He told his story to all of their members in the hopes
that it would help them take preventative measures, as
well as taking the threat of cancer seriously. A few years
after his first surgery, his cancer came back. He tried to go
a more natural route to healing the cancer, but ultimately
it killed him. I returned to South Bend to do consulting
work after Josh passed, and instead of Josh coming with

me to all of the classes, his wife went in his place. It took an immense amount of courage, but her presence alone spoke volumes to the firefighters. Josh had a YouTube channel where he and his kids would make silly videos. I will link one at the bottom that truly captures the essence of who Josh was.

https://www.youtube.com/watch?v=HrWEBtDJg9o&t=124s

When I became the wellness coordinator, my main goal was to not add any more names onto my leg. The legacy and face of each man is seared onto my heart, and their names are a permanent reminder to be grateful for each day that I live.

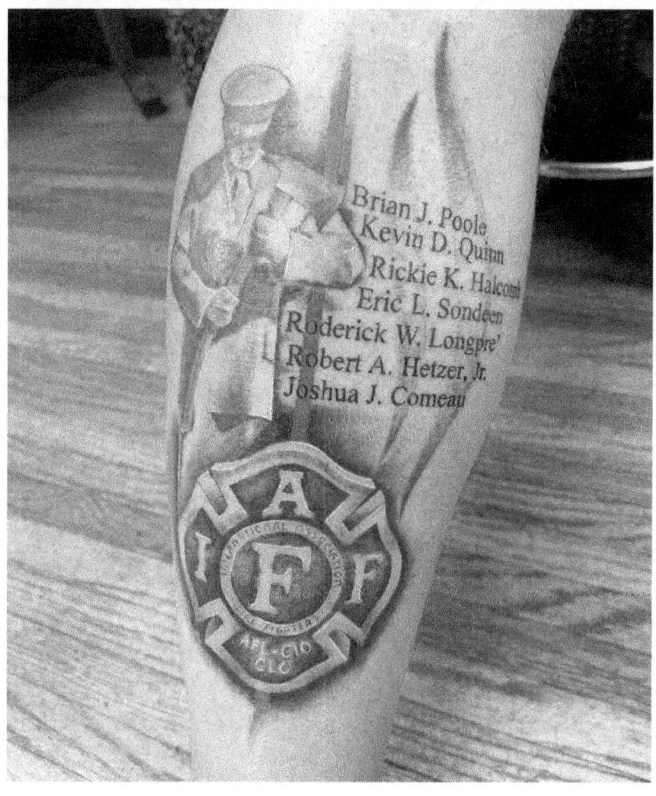

My tribute to my fallen friends

32 – THE AVENGERS

"There was an idea...To bring together a group of remarkable people to see if they could become something more."
-Nick Fury – The Avengers

I'd found a way for me to honor the fallen, but I'd be presented with a challenge to protect the living. It began one day when I received an intriguing message from the wife of a firefighter, who lived out of state. She claimed that our fire gear had perfluorooctanoic acid (PFOA) chemicals in them, which are known carcinogens. There are two large gear manufacturers in Dayton where I live, so I reached out to them for information about why PFOA would be in our gear. The manufacturers said there were only trace amounts, and those were only in legacy gear (gear created before 2015). I've been wearing fire gear since 1998, so I wasn't thrilled to hear that I'd been wearing gear that was tainted with even trace amounts of these harmful chemicals.

I didn't pursue the issue any further, assuming that if it were a real problem, the IAFF or the National Fire Protection Association (NFPA) would've addressed it. The woman who'd reached out to me on behalf of her firefighter husband was able to get in touch with Dr. Graham Peaslee, a scientist who works at the University of Notre Dame. She sent him her husband's gear to be tested. Dr. Peaslee found that there were *large* amounts of PFOA on the gear. PFOA is just one chemical out of more than 10,000 that are commonly known as Polyfluoroalkyl substances (PFAS), or forever chemicals. The term "forever chemicals" means the chemicals don't go away on their own. PFAS is commonly found in water repellants, non-stick cookware, (commonly called Teflon) fire gear, and firefighting foams.

The Last Call Foundation funded a study where thirty sets of fire gear were tested. PFAS was found on *all* the sets. Even with this groundbreaking information coming to light, the NFPA stayed radio silent.

The IAFF were given false information from a researcher who'd been bought and paid for by a gear manufacturer. A few years later, the IAFF funded their own study, which was consistent with the others, showing PFAS on the gear. Newly-elected president of the IAFF, Ed Kelly (Edzo), made it his mission to get rid of the harmful chemicals in the gear.

Gear manufacturers knew their gear contained harmful carcinogens and misled everyone by omitting that pertinent information. The gear manufacturers also had the support of the chemical companies, who were clearly choosing *profit* over the *health* of firefighters. When I started publicly speaking out against what they were doing, I didn't exactly make friends with the employees at local gear manufacturers. Living in the same small town, we'd run into each other frequently. To say that it was awkward is putting it lightly.

There was a small group of us gearing up to battle these manufacturers. We knew that they were bigger and more powerful than anything we could scrap together, hence the beginning of our squad, "The Avengers." These companies were a common threat to us, and the only chance we had at beating them was to band together. Individually, none of us wielded power or great influence. But together; we became a force to be reckoned with.

The ultraviolet (UV) test was the NFPA's standard test for our gear. In this test, the moisture barrier must be exposed to UV light for forty hours without disintegrating. The part of the fire gear they tested was inside the gear, which is never exposed to sunlight. It didn't make any sense to us. We wanted some clarification on this test, but the only answer we got was that the UV light test originated from a student thesis at the University of Kentucky. We called the library and requested a copy, but they told us that there are no digital copies available; the only copy that exists is a single hard copy in the University's student library.

It was no coincidence that I was off work recovering from my cancer surgery when we discovered this vital piece of information. Since I was the closest in proximity to Lexington and off work, I volunteered to make the drive and get a copy of the study. I called them to confirm they had a copy, and they told me that I was the third person to call about it, and that they were mailing it to North Carolina the following day. I told them I was on my way and asked them to make sure they didn't mail it yet. It felt as though I was in the *National Treasure* movie, vying for the treasure before the other side got ahold of it. The sense of urgency to get this hard copy in my hands increased with the knowledge that there were other people calling, also trying to obtain the study.

When I got to the library and found the study, it felt as if I'd struck gold. The Avengers and I celebrated like I was bringing home gold and diamonds—that's how valuable this report was to us. The copy proved that manufacturers were behind the study and knew that there were harmful chemicals in our gear. They chose to omit this information from the retailers who sold the gear. I wasn't just holding on to a copy of a student's thesis, I was holding a smoking gun. Our small group finally felt as though the tide had changed, we finally had a chance to win this thing. I went to make a copy of the report but found that the one printer in the entire University of Kentucky library was out of order. Fortunately, I was able to talk a student into logging me on to one of the library's computers that had a scanner attached. I was able to make what was believed at that time the first digital copy of this vital report.

Of course, magically, the next day, the NFPA found and emailed a digital copy of this study to everyone on their committee. The details to this study had been withheld from everyone, and the study was essentially a ghost—no one could produce it. Suddenly a digital copy appears after we found the hard copy? This kind of took the wind out of our sails, though it confirmed that someone was intentionally hiding information.

The IAFF picked up the baton and eventually sued the NFPA in an effort to get rid of the PFAS in our gear.

My old grade school and high school pal, Chad, worked for a company called Stedfast. It took about two years, but this company developed a moisture barrier for the gear that was able to pass the UV light test *without* any PFAS. It's funny to think about how Dayton played such an integral role in the grand scheme of things. The company that pushed for PFAS to be in our PPE was from Dayton, but Chad and I, also from Dayton, were able to come up with the solution to creating safe gear.

The opportunity to have fire gear that is free of PFAS should be available late 2023.

I'm currently on a committee with the IAFF that's working to create next generation PPE, free of toxic chemicals, that will keep firefighters safe while fighting fires.

It's very disheartening that gear meant to *protect* us contained detrimental carcinogens. It was an uphill battle, but our efforts were not in vain; new gear is in the process of being developed, and soon firefighters will no longer have to wear harmful gear.

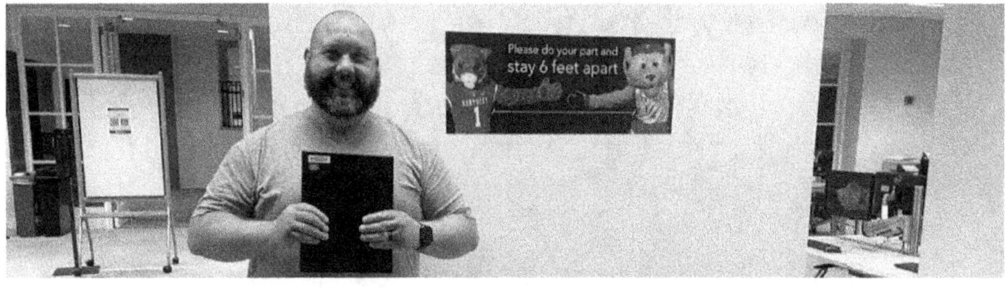

With the "Holy Grail" at the University of Kentucky library

"People raised on love see things differently than those raised on survival."
-Joe Marino

It was easy for me to jump into battle with the little guys against the big guys, but I struggled to acknowledge the battles raging within myself. The Save a Warrior (SAW) program gave me the opportunity to finally heal some of the inner turmoil I had buried for years.

Save a Warrior is an intervention program designed to help treat veterans, first responders, and active-duty military members suffering from childhood post-traumatic stress. I first heard about it through a friend of mine, and then it came up again in three interviews I did for my podcast. I was intrigued by the concept of it but really didn't know if it was for me. I knew I had some struggles, but I figured other people were worse off than I was, and I didn't want to take a seat away from them. I expressed this sentiment to a friend of mine who'd just returned from the program. He told me it wasn't really my place to decide that, and he encouraged me to leave that decision to those who were running the program.

I figured I didn't have anything to lose by applying, so I filled out an application and hit the *submit* button. They scheduled a phone interview with me, and Jake Wehr conducted my interview. I didn't hold back, peeling back a lot of layers and exposing my hidden addiction— food. I honestly thought other people didn't struggle with food addictions. In my job I see the results of drug and alcohol addictions, but never food. Jake told me that he also struggles with food addiction, and for the first time I didn't feel alone in my struggle.

SAW focuses on complex post-traumatic stress (PTS) from childhood. The program is built around the belief that your childhood experiences form and affect you as an adult. The way they determine the severity of your childhood trauma is through the Adverse Childhood Experiences (ACE) test. The test consists of ten questions and reflects exposure to a variety of household dysfunction or harmful experiences before the age of eighteen. The test questions are as follows:

Prior to your eighteenth birthday:

1.	Did a parent or other adult in the household often or very often... Swear at you, insult you, put you down, or humiliate you? or Act in a way that made you afraid that you might be physically hurt?
No___ Yes ___

2.	Did a parent or other adult in the household often or very often... Push, grab, slap, or throw something at you? or Ever hit you so hard that you had marks or were injured?
No___ Yes ___

3.	Did an adult or person at least five years older than you ever... Touch or fondle you or have you touch their body in a sexual way? or Attempt or actually have oral, anal, or vaginal intercourse with you?
No___ Yes ___

4.	Did you often or very often feel that ... No one in your family loved you or thought you were important or special? or Your family didn't look out for each other, feel close to each other, or support each other? No___ Yes ___

5.	Did you often or very often feel that ... You didn't have enough to eat, had to wear dirty clothes, and had no one to protect you? or Your parents were too drunk or high to take care of you or take you to the doctor if you needed it?
No___ Yes ___

6.	Were your parents ever separated or divorced?
No___ Yes ___

7.	Was your mother or stepmother ... Often or very often pushed, grabbed, slapped, or had something thrown at her? or Sometimes, often, or very often

kicked, bitten, hit with a fist, or hit with something hard? or Ever repeatedly hit over at least a few minutes or threatened with a gun or knife?
No___ Yes ___

8. Did you live with anyone who was a problem drinker or alcoholic, or who used street drugs?
No___ Yes ___

9. Was a household member depressed or mentally ill, or did a household member attempt suicide?
No___ Yes ___

10. Did a household member go to prison? No___ Yes ___

Add up your *yes* answers, and this is your ACE score. The higher your ace score, the higher your risk for social and health problems. According to the National Institute of Health, adults who had experienced four or more ACEs were twelve times more likely to be at risk of alcoholism, drug use, depression, and suicide attempts.

Based on my interview with Jake and my ACE score, I was accepted into the SAW program. On September 5, 2021, I drove to Hillsboro, Ohio, where I would stay for seventy-two hours and go through SAW's program. When I arrived, I looked around and soaked in the environment. It was beautiful, surrounded by serene woods and a lake.

I met the nine other guys who'd be going through the program with me. We were Cohort 0147, and over the next seventy-two hours, we'd build a bond that would typically take years to create. It was a heavy, deep three days, where we shared the unshareable, finally laying down burdens we had been carrying since childhood. Through our therapy sessions and bonfire conversations, no stone was left unturned. We spent a lot of time on the topic of forgiveness, both how to extend it and receive it.

We also focused on generational cycles and how to break them. When we are born into the world, we not only inherit a physical likeness to our parents, but we also inherit their narrative and deeply personal views. Transgenerational trauma refers to a kind of trauma that doesn't end with the individual and is passed on through generations. Many times, this is subtle and difficult to pinpoint. It can be something as small as negative coping mechanisms, to larger issues such as depression and addiction. We learned how to identify and break the chains that we've unknowingly been carrying.

I realized that my food addiction began as a comfort, a way to numb emotions. A child typically isn't going to crack open a beer, but a sleeve of Oreos sure made me feel better. This negative coping mechanism has followed me into adulthood. I knew I had to make changes, because it was a truly unhealthy path to be on.

Interestingly, at SAW, they encourage you to forgive people, but not necessarily reconcile with them. I can only speak for myself, but in my case, I wanted more than forgiving past transgressions. I wanted to resolve fractured relationships. This would eventually happen after more time and therapy.

I also made declarations while I was in SAW. In this sense a declaration is more than just a statement, it's your word and it's what you live by. These four declarations came from my heart without any rehearsing or prompting:

Love
Family
Leader
Honesty

I returned to SAW the following year, but this time in a different capacity. I came back to be what they call a shepherd, someone who helps guide the men going through the seventy-two-hour program. I didn't do anything significant in their program, instead did little things that helped them to be able to relax and solely focus on themselves and their recovery. I washed dishes, took out trash, and just helped where I could. It was pretty neat to go through the weekend in a different role, giving me a whole new perspective on the program.

In May of 2022, at the Ohio Association of Professional Firefighters (OAPFF) Conference in Cleveland, I spoke on a resolution I wrote on behalf of Dayton Firefighters Local 136, in which all career firefighters would contribute ten dollars over a two-year period to Save A Warrior. Save A Warrior had considerable donations from the veteran world, but hardly any funding from the first responder world. It was made clear to me that if first responders wanted the ability to attend SAW, they'd need to pony up some cash. I spoke in front of a couple hundred firefighters. Whatever speech I prepared was quickly thrown out for an opportunity to speak from the heart. I can't even recall what I said, but the next thing I know, several former SAW alumni I'd never met came to the mic and spoke about their positive experiences and how the program saved their lives. This was not planned; it's simply a reflection of how special and life-changing the program is. The president called for the vote and the resolution passed.

Later that day I received a text message from Jake Clark, the founder of SAW, which read, "It is never the masses who change history; rather, it is ALWAYS one man. Today, Jim . . . it's you. YOU did this. You stood for them. All of them. And we're proud to be your partner. You're that one man. Thank you so much for coming back for them, for us . . . it matters. You're changing the game and should feel SO proud. So much love."

He's right; I am proud of this resolution, and I'm proud of my fellow Ohio firefighters for supporting this cause.

I recommended this program to a lot of people who I thought could benefit from it. In turn, they went and then sent people close to them. We might not ever see the results of our actions, but it doesn't mean the connections aren't there. It was a ripple effect that I believe helped many hurting hearts find some solace.

For more information, please visit: https://saveawarrior.org

Source- https://cls.unc.edu/wp-content/uploads/sites/3019/2016/08/From-ACESTOOHIGH-ACES-and-Resilience-questions.pdf

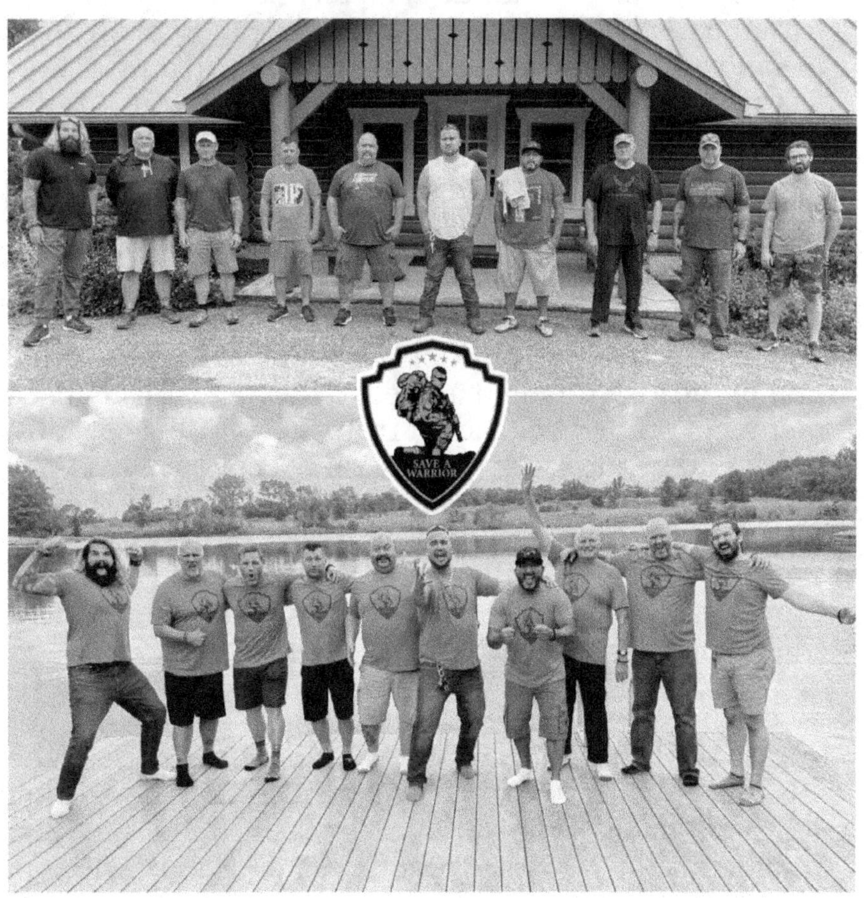

Cohort 0147 at SAW before and after our seventy-two hours

"Innovation is the ability to see changes as an opportunity, not a threat."
-Steve Jobs

Despite my efforts of working towards healing my mind, I continued to spiral after my cancer diagnosis. I'd begrudgingly returned to work after recovering from my cancer removal surgery. It seemed insane to jump right back into the environment that I believed caused my cancer, but I didn't really have another option. Imagine my happiness when the chief randomly texted me and asked me if I'd be interested in switching over to a forty-hour a week wellness coordinator position. I immediately responded with a resounding yes, without knowing any of the details. The chief thought that I would be a strong candidate for the position, and he recognized that the City of Dayton wasn't going to necessarily take care of us, so we'd have to be able to take care of our own.

I accepted the position without knowing the duration of the assignment. I agreed to the job knowing my members needed help, and I truly thought this new position could be the solution. After I'd been in it for a while, I was told the position was simply a trial they would explore for a period of three to six months. This information added an immense amount of pressure on me to try to prove that this position was critical to our members and should be a permanent position.

This was a brand-new position, and I was told to report to the assistant chief and work out the details of the job. Since this position had just been created, no one had a set layout of all of the duties and responsibilities the job would entail. We worked together to create feasible expectations for the position. I was ecstatic at the opportunity to work in this new position. I was physically and mentally burnt out, and this seemed like the perfect reset button. They had me set up my office in the fire headquarters, sharing an office with the fire marshall. (He had another office and was rarely at this one.) I had some concerns about the location of my office, knowing that the majority of firefighters wouldn't feel comfortable coming to see me at headquarters. The training center would have been a more preferable location, but I ultimately decided that I would go to the guys if they didn't feel comfortable coming to me.

I was super passionate about my new role and wanted to ensure I was focusing on the needs of the members in Dayton. I created an anonymous survey to collect data on the specific things our members were struggling with. It became apparent that the most pressing issues were suicide, depression, burnout, alcohol abuse and issues with sleeping. I think everyone assumed that I'd be mainly focused on cancer prevention, but I knew that I had to address these other issues first and foremost.

Initially, I had a lot of freedom to help the members as I saw fit. I felt as though I'd gained their trust, and I genuinely wanted to help them with their problems. It seemed as though I was making headway, and my bosses seemed happy with the progress we were making. I was only one person, but I felt I was making a positive impact with the members. Sometimes I would hit a wall with the assistant chief that I had to report to, but for the most part I didn't get discouraged.

I'd eventually realize that I wasn't heeding my own advice, and while I had the heart to help others through their struggles, I denied the existence of my own. I loved the position, but it was starting to take an enormous toll on me. My technical hours were from nine to five, but I often received late-night phone calls and texts from members, which I never ignored. It didn't matter what time someone contacted me, if they reached out, I'd do everything in my power to help them. I began to feel the pain of the people I was helping take root within my own body. I felt as though I was personally responsible for ensuring that no

one went through with their ideation of committing suicide. Due to confidentiality protocols, I had to be very
careful about what information I was allowed to share. I
took the privacy of the members seriously, and although
it's not their fault, their secrets began to weigh on me.
There were many times I felt too emotionally drained after helping others to ask those who were qualified for additional support. Some calls I received were heavy burdens I didn't want to place upon anyone else. I'm not a
small guy, but even *my* shoulders were crumbling beneath
the impossible weight I was attempting to bear.

35 – BEACON OF LIGHT

*"There are two ways of spreading light; to be the candle or the
mirror that reflects it."*
– Edith Wharton

When I became the wellness coordinator, I had all of the members take anonymous surveys regarding their mental health. An astounding amount of these surveys revealed that members were contemplating suicide or had thoughts of suicide in the past. This was terrifying to me; because the surveys were anonymous, I had no way of knowing who was in danger. It shook me that so many of our members were struggling with this serious issue. I wasn't sure what the solution was, but I knew we needed to address the pressing concern.

After the mass shooting in the Oregon District, Marathon Oil generously gave the union money to use towards enhancing mental health and wellness within the fire department. I thought that it would benefit our members to have someone from outside our organization come in. The union approved my idea, and I brought in Alison from Pinpoint Behavioral Health Center. She offered all members a checkup from the neck up while they were on duty. For the majority of my members, this was their first experience with a clinician.

I also convinced the city to bring in an outside speaker to talk about suicide. The fire department had never brought in an outside speaker during my tenure there. After discussing options with Lauren, it was clear who could shake the foundation of my Dayton fire members—Jo Terry. Jo's husband, Chip, was a firefighter for almost thirty years in Covington, KY. He struggled with undiagnosed post-traumatic stress injuries that led to his suicide. Chip left behind a loving wife, six children and one grandchild. Jo and Chip were married for thirty-one years, and she had no idea the internal battle he fought for years before ultimately succumbing to the pain. After his death, she made it her mission to help other families avoid losing a loved one who's dedicated their life to serving others. She's passionate about helping others avoid the devastating loss she's had to endure.

Both of these women agreed to come and teach classes to our members in the hopes of spreading mental health awareness and crushing the stigma of first responders asking for help. I set up a rigorous schedule, teaching twelve classes over a period of three days. Looking back, I shouldn't have scheduled so many classes. Jo is an incredibly effective speaker, but I didn't account for how painful it was for her to tell her story, over and over again. She did it for the sake of helping others, but it was a lot to ask of her. She's a champion for her cause, and our members benefited from her selflessness. Jo put the well-being of others above her own mental health. I can't speak for her, but I understand that sometimes preventing others from experiencing the trauma we've endured is worth the heartache it causes throughout the process.

There was a section in Jo's class where she listed the symptoms of post-traumatic stress. As she went over the symptoms, it was truly a lightbulb moment for my members. Some recognized that they were suffering from PTS and there was a good reason behind their undesirable behaviors. In every class, at least one person asked if we could do a class with spouses, to help explain why we (first responders) might behave the way we do. We ended up having two classes with members and their significant others. It was received well, and it is my opinion that our classes may have saved a few marriages.

Jo and Alison did an incredible job teaching the classes. We knew that there needed to be a shift in the culture of behavioral health and acknowledging the trauma we feel. We worked together to bring awareness and crush the stigma that only weak people ask for help.

It wasn't uncommon for people to stick around after class and ask questions, or even admit they weren't in a good headspace. There was one profound moment that stuck out to me, and it probably always will. After one class someone asked Jo if she's ever considered suicide, to which she promptly answered, "No."

The member replied, "I find it surprising that you've never thought of suicide."

Jo responded, "I find it surprising that you *have* thought of suicide. It's not normal to think that way."

The point she made landed a punch that I have never forgotten. She made the significant observation—so many people in our industry feel such intense pain that it isn't uncommon for suicide to cross their minds. Just because it isn't uncommon doesn't mean that it's healthy! Please, please don't take it lightly if you or someone you know thinks this is typical behavior. There are so many resources available to help you. Don't fall into the common trap of thinking that this could never happen to you or your loved ones. The harsh reality is that you'd be shocked if you knew who's found themselves contemplating suicide. It's very likely there are people in your circle who have been affected by suicidal ideation, either struggling with it themselves, or having a loved one who has. I know sometimes it seems as if the darkness will never fade, but the truth is that sometimes you have to break a little to let the light in. Thank you, Jo and Alison, for being a beacon of light in a dark world.

For more information on the Chip Terry Fund: https://www.thechipterryfund.org

For more information on Pinpoint Behavioral Health Center: https://www.pinpointbhs.com

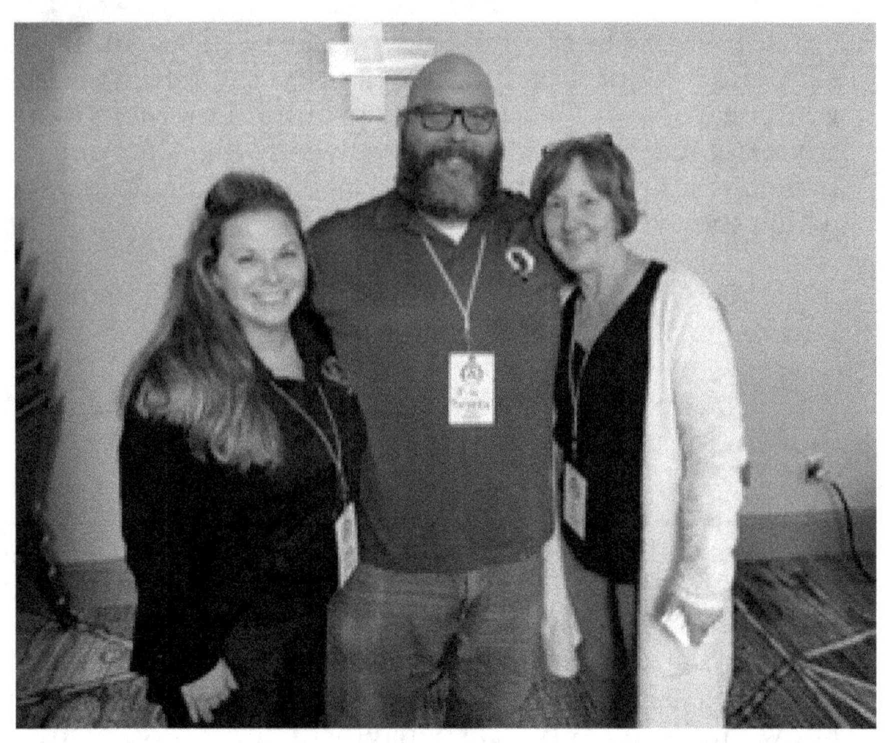

Alison, Me, and Jo at the First Responders Bridge Retreat
in Dublin Ohio

36 – EMERGENCY ROOM TERROR

*"Human beings are never going to be perfect. The best we can do
is to keep asking for help and accepting it when you can. And if
you keep on doing that, you'll always be moving towards better."*
-Leslie Higgins – Ted Lasso

As the peer support coordinator and the wellness coordinator, I was able to help people all over the area. Although firefighters were my priority, if police needed additional support, I was always happy to help them. As I've mentioned, I've been called to some pretty serious and awful situations. When there's an event so traumatic first responders have difficulty processing what they just experienced, that's where we jump in. Our team wasn't limited in only helping police officers and firefighters. One horrific night we were even called to the hospital to offer peer support to doctors and nurses.

It was common practice for a sheriff to accompany an inmate to the hospital if they needed to receive medical attention. One night there was an inmate who was receiving treatment in the emergency room. A sheriff accompanied him and then passed him off to an armed security guard hired through a private security company. The security guard that was in the room with the inmate was seventy-eight years old and walked with the assistance of a cane. No one knows exactly what happened, but there was a struggle between the inmate and the security guard. The inmate was able to overtake the security guard and steal his gun. He shot and killed the security officer in the small hospital room.

Then the prisoner erratically ran from the room in an attempt to escape the hospital, wildly pointing the gun at everyone in his path. Doctors and nurses scrambled out of his way, having heard the shots fired. The man made it outside to the hospital entrance where he proceeded to kill himself.

You can imagine the hysteria and panic happening inside the emergency room department. Nurses were used to patients being somewhat aggressive at times, but there were metal detectors at the entrance of the emergency room. A weapon wasn't a threat hospital staff typically had to worry about.

My team met with the doctors and nurses who had been in the emergency room during the shooting. They were understandably traumatized. A lot of them changed departments following this incident; it ruined the safe sanctuary of their job. The hallways were no longer safe places, and the rooms were tainted with the death of the security guard. One man had taken their peace and security away from them.

I'm proud of the work our team did, and the fact that no one questioned jumping in to help the hospital staff. Post-traumatic stress (PTS) is not unique to firefighters and police officers. I firmly believe that ALL first responders need someone to advocate for them. We are all helpers, fighting on the same team. No one can take that away from us.

37 – THE BEGINNING OF THE END

"Life can only be understood backwards; but it must be lived forwards."
-Soren Kierkegaard

I took my peer support work very seriously, and I was getting settled into my wellness coordinator role. As time went on, I recognized that the fire department needed to make some pretty significant changes. One of the main things I lobbied for was a policy change regarding the treatment and expectation of members after going on traumatic calls. Imagine going on a run where there is a violent death or horrific accident. As a first responder, sometimes you witness the worst in humanity. You finish the call and are expected to jump right into the next one, with a clear head. I knew firsthand how flawed the system was, so I pushed for a policy change that allowed members to *immediately* meet with a clinician after a traumatic event, or even clock out and go home, allowing them to process what they'd just experienced. However, this policy was not approved by the assistant chief.

As wellness coordinator, my main priority was suicide prevention. I was doing everything in my power to support our members. One of my biggest fears happened when I received a text during dinner one night, saying that there was a BOLO out on one of our members, Brandon, and he intended to kill himself. It took me a minute to wrap my head around Brandon being in this position. He was the type of guy that everybody liked. He was smart and kind. Brandon was in the annual firefighter fundraiser calendar, and this dude's muscles had muscles. He was young and had the world at his fingertips.

Brandon had just finished working a shift during which he encountered two horrific calls; to say he was in a bad headspace doesn't even touch his mental state. We sprang into action, searching for him and following up on leads until around midnight. All of the leads we chased were dead ends. Defeated, exhausted, and imagining the worst, we called it a night.

When I woke up the next morning, I saw that the police had pinged his car, and they'd located it at an abandoned church. He wasn't in his car, so the search for him continued. No one knew if he'd be dead or alive when he was finally found.

I went to the firefighter activity center to reach out to peer support for the members. I received a text saying that Brandon had been found dead. The grief I felt was overwhelming, but I was in protector mode, so I made calls to get grief counselors and clinicians out to the activity center. Eleven minutes after receiving the text about his death, I got a text with conflicting information, that his death was not confirmed and the manhunt was still underway. He was found an hour later, in very bad shape, but *alive.*

At this point, there were so many versions of the story going around, no one knew what to believe. When you were a kid did you ever play the game Telephone? You whisper a phrase to the person next to you, and they say it to the person next to them, and so forth. By the time the message gets to the last person, it's always completely different from the original phrase. The same thing happened here, but instead of a silly message, it was dire information regarding the life of a beloved friend. I had coordinated support at the union hall and asked permission for crews that were struggling to come and talk to someone there. It was an emotional roller coaster, and the members were deeply impacted. The assistant chief denied my request, so because they couldn't come to us, I turned on the bat signal and called in peer supporters from the region to visit the on-duty Dayton crews.

Brandon was in critical condition in the ICU, and when he was stable enough, he was moved to the mental health floor. It would take several more weeks before

Brandon started to remember anything from this incident. I was able to set up reservations for him to attend the IAFF Center of Excellence. He was alive, but he had a long road of recovery ahead of him. This should've been comforting to me, but I couldn't shake the reality of what had almost happened. It was a near miss, my worst nightmare. That night, sleep evaded me, so I tried to work out. Suddenly I was uncontrollably sobbing, the grief, exhaustion, and fear finally surfacing and leaving my body. I was trying so hard to make sure that everyone else was taken care of that I neglected to allow myself to process what had happened.

In the midst of trauma, your response is typically not perfect. Some people thought that I went too far by going to the stations and offering help. It's easy to look back on a situation and see what you could have done better. I was continuing to learn how to navigate in this role, and it was taking a huge emotional toll on me. This story will never leave me for various reasons—one being it was the beginning of when I started to unravel.

The week after the near miss, I had a meeting with the assistant chief. I was still riding an emotional roller coaster. I took the week off work, knowing that I wasn't in any position to be able to perform my job. I hadn't shaved, had circles under my eyes that showed my exhaustion, and I was wearing a casual outfit for the meeting.

The second I walked through the door, the negative tone to the meeting was set when the deputy chief sarcastically asked me, "Is that the new uniform?"

I curtly replied, "I don't know, is *that* the new uniform?" (referring to his Miami-Vice looking suit). Already on edge, the comment pushed me over. I entered the assistant chief's office and shut the door, and what should've been a calm and productive meeting turned into frustration boiling over into seething anger. I blamed the assistant chief for our near miss, feeling that if the policy I'd been trying to get approved was in place, Brandon would've likely had a different outcome after enduring two back-to-back traumatic calls.

We were supposed to have a meeting with HR regarding the traumatic call policy, and the assistant chief made the executive decision that it would be best if he took the meeting without me. Both of our emotions were running so high that I agreed with him. I was too close to the issue to remain impartial and not get emotional in the meeting.

The following Saturday, I was having dinner at Texas Roadhouse before a Garth Brooks concert in Cincinnati, when I got a text saying that one of our guys, Andy, was in a situation. Walking away from warm Texas Roadhouse rolls to deal with another issue was frustrating for my wife and our friends who met us for dinner. It was becoming very evident that I was always on call, and I should just forget any plans I'd made. Fortunately, another member on the peer support team was able to meet with Andy and help him out. Even with the quick assistance, this situation would come back to haunt me a few days later. Andy had lied about what had transpired between him and the peer supporter he met with. Although Andy had a reputation for dishonesty, *my* reputation would be the one put on the line.

There were sure to be ramifications from my heated meeting with the assistant chief. Although my emotions were justifiable, my anger directed towards him could easily be viewed as a form of insubordination. I was on the peer support team, as well as the sole wellness coordinator for my department. The stress of the job was growing with each call for help I received. The path I was on was not sustainable, but I willed myself to forge ahead, one foot in front of the other. I wouldn't realize it until it was too late, but each step was taking me a little closer to my demise.

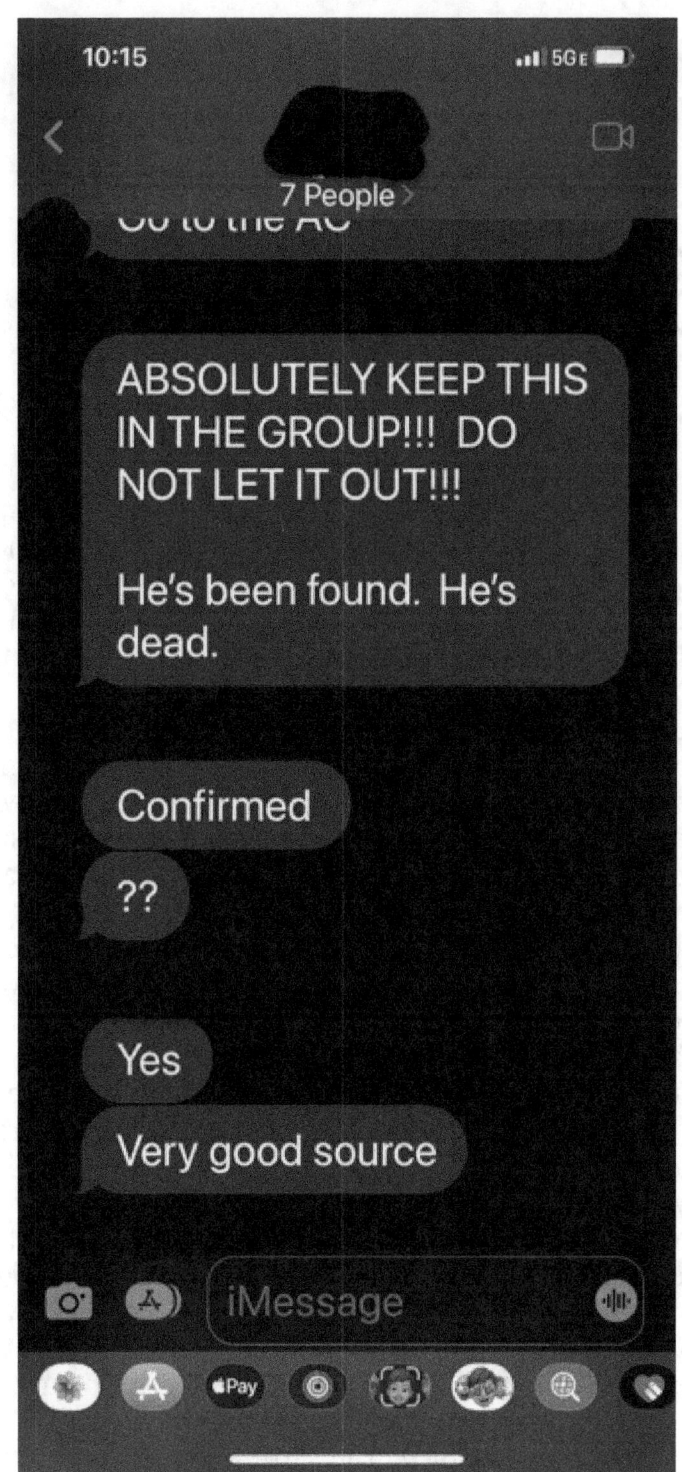
10:15
7 People
ABSOLUTELY KEEP THIS IN THE GROUP!!! DO NOT LET IT OUT!!!

He's been found. He's dead.
Confirmed
??
Yes
Very good source
iMessage

38 – CLEVELAND DOESN'T ROCK

*"The bravest thing I ever did was continuing my life when I
wanted to die."*
-Juliette Lewis

Boomer and I were heading to Cleveland to attend an OAPFF conference. We were both looking forward to escaping the chaos at home. The near miss with Brandon and then the situation with Andy weighed heavily on us, but they were both alive, so we felt as though we could finally breathe.

Boomer and I made it to Cleveland, and I got a call regarding Andy, who had been helped by a member on our peer support team while I was at the Garth Brooks concert. Andy claimed that his confidentiality had been breached by the peer supporter who met with him. (I later had a conversation with Andy and the peer supporter and concluded that his confidentiality had not been violated. Andy has since resigned in lieu of being fired from the fire department for *lying* and drinking on the job.) However, although there was no truth to his claim, it still resulted in me being investigated by the department, as well as the union. I was in shock. I had a solid reputation, but my integrity and character were in question after one bogus claim. I didn't need a pat on the back, but blame was misplaced on my shoulders. I was experiencing organizational betrayal after merely following protocol. Boomer was so taken aback by the news that he resigned from the peer support team, effective immediately. I started spiraling. Boomer was my right-hand man, and even *with* him the job wasn't sustainable. There was no way I could continue to work in my position without additional support. Desperate for a lifeline, I called the assistant chief and explained that I was feeling overwhelmed and betrayed by the very department for which I had sacrificed so much in order to give my all. I told him I needed help, and he responded "I don't have time to help you." I couldn't believe that I was being gaslit by the same guys I was fighting for.

This wasn't the first time I'd been morally injured, but it cut the deepest.

The real punch landed when I learned that Brandon had been sent to the ER due to Diabetic Ketoacidosis (DKA). Brandon's sugar was out of whack, and he'd thrown up all over the bunk room at the Center of Excellence (COE). Brandon decided that he wouldn't be returning to the COE after he was released from the hospital. Everyone else that I'd sent there successfully completed the program and returned home in a healthy mental state. I hadn't experienced someone leaving before completing the program. I felt confident that he was safe at the COE, but now that he was no longer in their care, my fear and anxiety began ramping up.

I went to bed feeling vulnerable and alone. I woke up in the middle of the night to a voice saying, "Hey, suicide is an option." I was groggy and confused, as I didn't recognize this voice. It didn't let up. As a concealed carry holder, I'd had a gun stolen out of my truck once, so as a precaution, I'd brought it up to my hotel room. The voice reminded me that my gun was a few feet away. I could quickly and easily put an end to all the pain I was feeling.

I walked over to my gun, contemplating what I should do. I know it sounds crazy, but looking back, I believe I was experiencing intense mental and spiritual warfare. The voice was relentless, tempting me to end it all. I thought about my two boys and my wife and snapped out of the groggy haze I was stuck in. I took the magazine out of the gun, and I placed them in two separate drawers. The rest of the night, I tried turning off the voice, but I couldn't. I felt sick with fear and anxiety. I was exhausted the next day, but I was too ashamed and embarrassed to tell anyone what had happened. My main priority and factor of stress was preventing suicide, and here I was, contemplating it. I felt like a fraud. My pride kept me from confiding in Boomer, and I know without a doubt he would've helped me. I had to just pretend as if I was okay.

Somehow, I made it through the rest of the trip without anyone noticing that something was off with me.

I narrowly escaped ending my life, but I knew I wasn't in the clear. The strange voice I heard that night had not left me. I didn't want to risk a repeat of what happened in the hotel room back when I was home. As soon as I got back in town, I called my friend Bryan and simply said, "I have something in a bag that I need to give you." I didn't have to say what the bag contained, or why I needed to give it to him to hold on to. He knew what I wasn't saying. He left work and met me at a gas station, taking the gun without any questions. I haven't seen it since.

The gun was out of my possession, but the voice didn't disappear, continuing to taunt me. I didn't tell anyone what had happened, not even Lauren or my family. Like all of the other bad things I've endured, I shoved it down and tried to ignore it. This was too loud and big for me to ignore for long. I talked to a clinician, but it would be months before I admitted that I needed help. I knew how serious this was, but I couldn't let anyone know how I was feeling. After all, I was the wellness guy—only I was far from well. There wasn't a script or camera, but my acting debut had begun.

"Fake happiness is the worst kind of sadness."
-Dominic Riccitello

A local news station was doing a story on post-traumatic stress disorder PTSD in First Responders. Steve Click, the director of the Ohio Office of First Responder Wellness, reached out to see if I had any interest in giving an interview for the story. As the wellness coordinator, I was happy to help bring awareness to the growing problem of PTSD in first responders.

The department gave me the green light to be interviewed on behalf of Dayton Local 136, with the caveat that someone accompany me to ensure I stayed in line. I'd been known to go a little rogue, and not too long before had made noise about the city and their lack of support for firefighters battling cancer. You could say I was a little bit of a risk; no one ever knew what was going to come out of my mouth, myself included. My friend Brad played chaperone while I met with the reporters and gave the interview.

During the interview, I talked about the slow evolution of behavioral health in our culture and work environment. I talked about how when I first started on the job, it was taboo to talk about feelings or things with which we struggled, but that we were starting to see the tide turn and recognize that we needed to change the culture and bring awareness to the growing epidemic of first responders struggling with depression and post-traumatic stress (PTS). I said that it's imperative that people process trauma in a healthy way and get help early on. We talked about the various resources available to help first responders who are struggling. There's a line I said that didn't seem very significant at the time, but would resonate in my sister for months after hearing it. I said "You know, we're used to seeing a ton of traumatic events that the normal person maybe sees once or twice in a lifetime . . . and for us it's just a day. It's Tuesday for us." It struck a chord in her because that short sentence spoke volumes about the daily trauma we experience. It opened her eyes to the reality that the horrific calls we experience merely blend in with the rest of our days.

The truly crazy thing about this interview is that I was struggling with immense inner turmoil while giving it. Here I was, circling the drain, yet offering advice on how and where to seek help if needed. I was being such an enormous hypocrite. I talked about breaking the stigma and helpers asking for help, yet I couldn't bring myself to do it. That is how powerful the hold of the fear of judgment can grip someone. Internally, I was self-destructing, yet talking about how we were changing the narrative on getting help when struggling.

To give you a picture of where I was at mentally and emotionally when I gave this interview, it was done on July 7th, 2022. I checked myself into the Center of Excellence (COE) on August 20th, 2022. This interview is a prime example of my acting. I hid behind the mask I grew comfortable wearing, for about a month after this interview, until even the mask couldn't conceal the turmoil I had been enduring.

When I was at the COE, I had very limited time on my phone. My family and friends (who knew where I was) were left baffled, trying to understand how one minute I was fine and the next suddenly in crisis-mode. Because I acted as if I was fine for way longer than I should have, they were left in a state of confusion. My sister wrote a song called "Tuesday" that helped her process it all. I'm sharing it here because I think she was able to capture the emotions I was feeling. The song was inspired by the recent interview I had given, specifically the quote above where I referenced a tragic day just being another "Tuesday" for us:

Tuesday

No one talks about the bad days,
They just cover up their heartache.
Assume it's all good but instead,
Hanging on by a thread . . .

You look fine on the outside,
They think you're okay.
Cause' no one can see,
A heart break.
Tired of fighting,
Praying for change.
But life goes on like,
It's just Tuesday.

People are laughing,
And I wonder when,
The last time I laughed,
And will I do it again.
Hustle and grind the world screams,
But I can't seem to move my feet.

You look fine on the outside,
They think you're okay.
Cause' no one can see,
A heart break.
Tired of fighting,
Praying for change.
But life goes on like,
It's just Tuesday.

I just keep driving,
With nowhere to go.
Trying not to feel,
So lost and alone.
Hoping to leave some pieces behind,
Pick up all the peace that I can find.

You look fine on the outside,

They think you're okay.
Cause' no one can see,
A heart break.
Tired of fighting,
Praying for change.
But life goes on like,
It's just Tuesday.

Eyes can't unsee
A heart can't unfeel
Pretending it didn't happen,
Won't make it unreal.
Hope my tears won't always last,
There's no way to change the past.

But it won't stay Tuesday,
It's gonna be alright.
Let out the pain
Let in the light.
Together we'll get through
All of this rain.
And tomorrow it won't be . . .
Tuesday.

It cannot stay Tuesday. As first responders, there's no way to shield ourselves from trauma and tragedy. That's the nature of a lot of calls to which we respond. But we can process the trauma in a healthy way. We can vocalize how we feel after returning from a terrible call. There are various therapies we can participate in to help with the more difficult things. There's no good reason to stay stuck in the mindset that the things we encounter are normal; they are far from normal.

If I went into a fire and broke my leg, I'd go to the hospital and get my leg treated. I'd use crutches to walk, and no one would think anything of it. So why is it when we injure our brains during a call, we're afraid to seek treatment? A brain injury is probably more serious, yet is ignored, time and time again. If I was limping around with a broken leg, you'd say I was crazy and urge me to go to the doctor. But when I walk around with an injured brain, I'm applauded and called *brave*. It has got to stop! *Any* injury deserves medical attention without judgement.

We also need to stop comparing our pain. There are such a wide variety of terrible calls we go on, and we can't compare the level of trauma we endured with our assumption of what a different crew experienced on another scene. It is like comparing a bite to a sting. They are two different types of pain, but *they both still hurt*! It's not up to us to say which hurts more or which is worse. There's a certain level of this in the first-responder world. People don't want to be sympathetic when they've been on a similar run multiple times. It doesn't negate the fact that there's still trauma involved with the call! We've got to crush the stigma that keeps us from seeking help, and together, get beyond Tuesday.

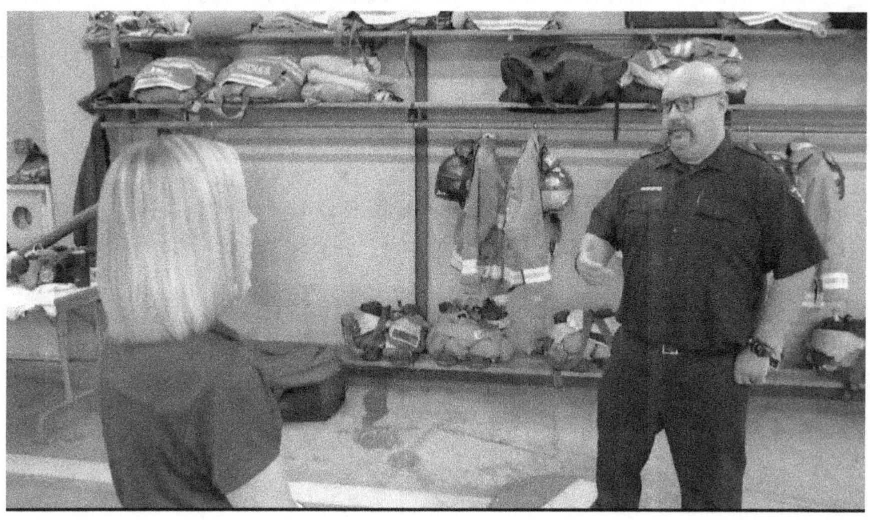

Faking my way through an interview with Channel 2 about PTSD in first responders

40 – MAN IN THE MIRROR

"You are imperfect, you are wired for struggle, but you are worthy of love and belonging."
-Brene Brown

I want to describe in detail what it looked like at the height of my anxiety and depression. These mental illnesses are not one-size-fits-all, and symptoms vary from person to person. I can only speak candidly about what I experienced.

For me, the depression made the act of getting out of bed a chore that seemed overwhelming most days. Something I'd never had to think twice about felt like an impossible task. All I wanted to do was lie in my bed and sleep. I had zero motivation to do anything. Through my counseling sessions, I learned that while some just sleep excessively, others dissociate from their life. This includes their job, family, friends, and activities that they used to enjoy.

I stopped caring about my physical health. All of the healthy habits I'd worked towards creating were crushed. My only other source of comfort when not sleeping was eating. When I was awake, I ate all kinds of food, regardless of if I was hungry or not. I gained about fifty pounds over the course of three or four months. I completely stopped working out. Getting out of bed was draining enough. I couldn't muster the physical energy necessary to exercise. I lost the mental capacity to take care of myself, or anyone else, for that matter.

The anxiety I experienced was crippling. It was as if the depression led me to my bed, and the anxiety kept me chained to it. My bedroom was my only safe haven. I missed out on so many things I cared about due to my anxiety, including my kids' sports practices and games; activities I used to love to watch. I wasn't showing up for my family or anyone, for that matter. It wasn't because I didn't want to; I physically couldn't will my body to move.

My thought process was pretty much that if I didn't leave my house, nothing out of my control or bad would happen to me. My sleep was super erratic. There were a lot of nights that I couldn't sleep, so I would go in to work early and try to distract myself from the thoughts that would enter my mind. My goals were to avoid people, events, and my thoughts. This went on for months.

I didn't realize I was suffering from post-traumatic stress disorder (PTSD). For me, this included agitation, depression, anxiety, and hypervigilance. I made rash decisions that did not come from a logical, sound place. They were made out of irrational fear.

The most frustrating part of this was that although my brain was sick, it was an invisible sickness. There was no telltale rash or fever that alerted others that I was unwell. There were no visible bruises or scars on my skin, though my heart was broken. There was no physical evidence other than my weight gain and tendency to oversleep that I was suffering from mental health issues. If I were to look in the mirror, I couldn't see anything that was happening in my heart or head. There were no signs of the brokenness in which I was operating. I looked just like myself. It's dangerous, because if I can't see it in my own reflection, no one else around me can see it either. I hid these debilitating thoughts from my closest friends and family for months. The image I saw in the mirror was not a clear picture of who I was, just a reflection of the lies I told.

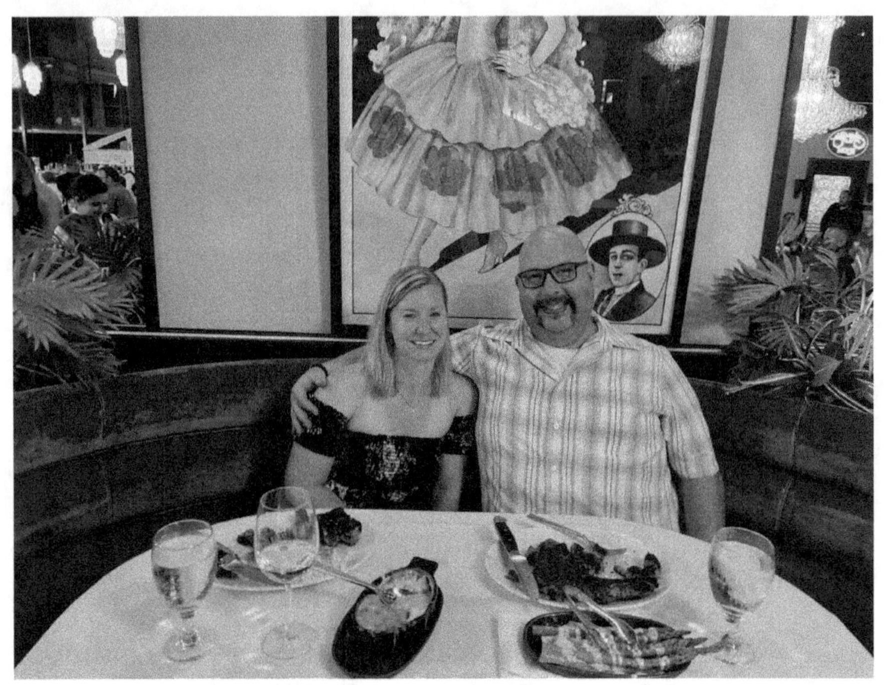

One week before I finally admitted that I needed help.

41 – IT'S A FAMILY OATH

"If there is no struggle, there is no progress."
-Frederick Douglass

For a long time, I was too ashamed to tell my loved ones that I was suffering, and completely understand the fear that accompanies letting walls down. However, it's crucial to communicate your struggles with your significant other. Their support is imperative throughout the healing process.

There are two conferences that Lauren and I attended that I highly recommend for first responders and their spouses. These conferences help shed light on the issues that commonly come with the job. They provide a window into the world that first responders live in, giving insight into common problems (PTS, anxiety, depression, suicidal ideation) that we might struggle with. A lot of this wasn't initially on my radar, so I want to share some common signs and symptoms people may exhibit when experiencing some of these mental health issues. Some symptoms of PTS include agitation, isolation from loved ones, fear, anxiety, and nightmares. Anxiety symptoms include restlessness, fatigue, increased heart rate and a sense of panic. Signs of depression may include apathy, anxiety, sadness, fatigue, irritability/moodiness, extreme weight gain or weight loss, and isolation. Warning signs of someone having suicidal thoughts include people talking about wanting to die, feeling as if they are a burden to others, feeling hopeless, isolating themselves from loved ones, extreme moodiness, and eating and sleeping significantly more or less. It helps to understand some of the symptoms associated with mental health issues in order to help a loved one who may be experiencing them.

I can tell you from personal experience that a lot of the time, our significant others are left in the dark regarding the traumatic calls we respond to. What they get instead is the aftermath of the call—our unexplained moods and emotions or the symptoms of a bigger issue, such as PTS or depression. This can lead to a lot of frustration and disagreements. There's a high divorce rate among first responders. It's important to be proactive in your marriage and become intentional about communication with your spouse. I've been guilty of wanting to protect Lauren, so I wouldn't talk to her about certain hard calls I'd gone on. In the long run, this behavior only hurt both of us.

The First Responders' Bridge is a well put together educational and informative retreat for first responders and their significant others. They typically accept over one hundred couples at each conference. It's a two-day conference covering a large span of information that's very helpful in giving spouses a glimpse into the world their first responders live in, as well as a clue in the first responders to the perspective of their significant others. They do not charge admission as their goal is to help those who've experienced life-altering or traumatic events.

Ohio ASSIST Post Critical Incident Seminar (PCIS) is another helpful conference that Lauren and I attended. Ohio ASSIST is a smaller, more intimate conference, with only around thirty couples. This conference is more interactive and gives couples the opportunity to talk to clinicians and process their problems in a healthy and safe environment. This is a free program as well that provides counseling, education, and peer support for first responders.

I met Lisa Taylor here, who unfortunately suffered through horrible organizational betrayal. I had gone through this as well but didn't know there was an actual name for this form of deception. After talking to Lisa, it became clear to me that I needed to address this problem. When it was my turn to sit down with a clinician, this was the main issue I focused on throughout the conference.

I did EMDR regarding the Workman incident and how I was treated after it happened. When I gave everything to my job and the people I was working with, I just couldn't wrap my mind around how poorly I was treated afterwards. Lauren sat down with a clinician and did EMDR as well, regarding me and how abruptly I left to go to the Center of Excellence. The crisis I was facing inadvertently threw Lauren into crisis mode as well. Overnight, without warning, she was thrown into the role of a single mom for forty days. I am grateful that Lauren was given the opportunity to receive some help regarding the issues she carried as a result of my actions.

This past December, I returned to the Bridge Retreat, but this time around I was a peer supporter, helping others. It was pretty incredible to witness things come full circle. I'm grateful that I had the chance to pay it forward and help someone who might be stuck in the same place I was last year. We can't change what we experienced in the past, but we *can* determine how to move forward towards healing.

42 – WHAT THE ARMOR CAN'T COVER

"Sometimes hitting rock bottom is the best thing that ever happened to you. Because you go running back to what you know, and you take inventory of everything in your life, and you start from scratch."
-Drew Barrymore

I'd been working on a grant proposal that would pay for my wellness coordinator position, ensuring that I could stay on and continue to help the members. I was gaining their trust and picking up momentum in my quest against crushing the stigma of getting help. In my proposal, the grant would also include retention bonuses for firefighters. I thought this would be a great incentive to stay with the department, as we were losing members at a high rate due them being overworked and miserable.

Shortly after returning home from the OAPFF conference in Cleveland, my office was moved from the headquarters to the training center. I thought it would be a move that benefitted me; members would be more likely to come see me at the training center than they would at headquarters. I would be reporting to a new boss, allowing me to have a little more freedom to do my job.

I had one last falling out with my previous chief regarding peer support. I told him he wasn't following the policy moving forward with peer support. When he failed to commit to adhere to the policy, I told him my next step would be to get the union involved. He told me if I got the union involved, I'd find myself back on the street in my old position. I should've been surprised that my position was being threatened, but after all that I'd been through, it seemed par for the rocky road I'd been on.

I had a meeting with my new boss, an assistant chief that I was excited to work with. I was hopeful he'd be a little more receptive to what I was trying to accomplish and help me accrue the necessary resources to become successful. However, all of those hopes were dashed in our first meeting, when he told me that I had lost my position. I was no longer the health and wellness coordinator; I was to resume my former position back on the street as a firefighter and medic.

This news caught me off guard and devastated me. I was finally making headway. I knew I didn't get it right all the time, but my team was making a positive impact on a lot of members. I felt as though I was someone they could come to without being judged, and genuinely had a heart for wanting to help them. But all of that was gone in one meeting. Every minute of lost sleep, time away from my family, tears cried, all of it gone for no good reason. I had found my purpose through this position; without the job, I felt as though I no longer had purpose. I had inner turmoil that I tried my best to disguise; after all, I'd been acting for so long, this would be yet another scene I had to fake my way through.

I still had a few more weeks in my wellness coordinator position before I was due back at the firehouse. I was in my office, when, for the first time, I was called out on my state of mind by a good friend who wasn't fooled by my act. He pulled back the curtain and blatantly told me what I was doing wasn't healthy, and if I didn't make a change, they would be adding *my* name to the memorial of fallen firefighters. It was the perfect opportunity to tell him that he was right and ask for help. But I didn't admit to needing, nor did I ask for help. The fracture in my armor exposed, the whole thing started to crack. I carried on my act, knowing I couldn't keep up the role much longer. I messaged my captain and told her I wasn't coming back. I was going to burn through my sick leave while awaiting my return to the district. It was during that week-and-a-half off that I started to admit I was struggling. I reached out and started attending a local first responder intensive outpatient program (IOP). Although it's a great program, it was too little too late. I was too broken, too far gone, for it to work for me.

I was supposed to go back to the firehouse on a Monday, so the Friday before, I bitterly cleaned out my office and transported my things to Station 8. The reality of my situation sank in as I put my belongings in the station; and in that moment I knew I could not do it.

My parents were watching my boys, and Lauren and I were going to go see Chris Stapleton in concert that evening. We were both excited to see him, though we never made it there. I went to pick up the boys from my parents' house, and I was talking to my mom on the porch when I got there. It was a long time coming, and I finally lost it. She asked me pointed questions, seeing I wasn't okay but not knowing how bad it truly was. It was as if all the tears I'd swallowed broke through the barrier I created, a flood of tears overflowing from my cut heart.

I was so upset I couldn't even drive myself or my kids home. My mom drove my boys to my house, and my dad drove me in my truck. Lauren arrived about the same time we did, taking in the scene and realizing that our life was about to change.

I knew there was only one place where I had a chance to heal. I told Lauren I needed to get myself in to the Center of Excellence, and she supported me and told me she'd handle everything at home and gave me her blessing to go. This was a really hard phone call to make, as ironically, I'd already made it five times for members I'd been helping. This time, when I called, I had to swallow my pride and tell the receptionist that I was calling for myself. That night was a whirlwind. I had one night to get all of my affairs in order, pack for a thirty to forty-five day stay, and spend what little time was left with my family. The next afternoon I would be on a flight to Maryland.

43 – Maryland

"Trust the process."
-Every employee at the Center of Excellence

After making a call the night before, I found myself on an airplane heading to Maryland so I could attend the IAFF Center of Excellence Treatment Center (COE). The last-minute decision was stressful, causing me to rush around as I packed my belongings and tied up loose ends before leaving. It was such a whirlwind that I don't think I had time to properly process what was happening until I was finally sitting on the plane. I came undone on the plane, sobbing the entire flight. I'm sure people thought I was crazy; *well, welcome to the club* is what I'd say to them. I was anxious about the journey ahead and felt guilty about leaving my family behind. Ultimately, I knew that, more than anyone else, they benefitted from a healthy version of me, a version I haven't been in quite some time.

There was an escort from the COE waiting for me at the airport, and he drove me to the center. The center was designed specifically to treat professional firefighters struggling with substance abuse, addiction, trauma, and/or other behavioral health issues. It is unique in the sense that every employee there understands the trauma and struggles that we face throughout our profession.

When I think of recovery or treatment centers, I think of all white, sterile walls with gates and fences to keep patients from leaving. This center couldn't be any further from that! It sits on fifteen acres of land, surrounded by lavish evergreen and pine trees. There are walking trails and places to sit outside to reflect and relax in nature. The trees and wooded areas are inviting and serene. There are four station houses where patients stay, and the design of each house is modeled after fire stations, giving patients a sense of familiarity. There are four beds to a room, similar to the set-up at firehouses. The center offers plenty of amenities, such as a basketball court, volleyball court, a swimming pool, and a fully equipped gym. There are no gates prohibiting anyone from leaving, as people attend on a voluntary basis.

One thing I liked about the program right off the bat is that people don't arrive at the same time, so patients are in different stages of recovery. I saw guys that were close to graduating the program, and they looked sincerely happy. It gave me genuine hope that at the end of my time, I would find the same level of joy they exuded.

I had to pass a Covid test to enter the facility, as we were still in the thick of the pandemic. My test came back negative, and Alex, who had just graduated and was getting ready to leave, asked me a simple question, "Are you a thinker or a drinker?" It made me laugh, as I'd never heard the question posed that way. I was in there because I was a thinker. I got settled in, hopeful and broken, wondering what was to come.

It was surreal to me how much had changed in a year. A year before I checked myself in to the COE, I sat down with a group of four guys that had successfully completed the program. We created a video of our conversation, where they shared their raw and honest experiences from the center. The COE uses this video to give insight into what it looks like going through their program, from the perspective of four men who had gone through it. One year ago, I was moderating a candid conversation, and now here I was, about to experience it all firsthand.

I already had it in my head that I was going to fast track this program, acing my way through the classes and therapy sessions. After all, I was the wellness coordinator for Dayton. I had served on the peer support team for a couple of years. I knew the right things to do, I just needed help applying them to myself. The average stay is about thirty-five days. I'd be out in thirty, just in time for our long-awaited Disney trip. We had been saving and planning for a long time for this trip. The boys were stoked; they'd never been to Disney before. The big kid in me was stoked to spend some quality time in the new *Star Wars* area. After what I was putting my family through in my absence, Lauren and the boys deserved the trip of a lifetime.

One day Alex asked me if I wanted to go to the worship service with him, and though my faith had waned through the years, I agreed. What I'd been doing clearly wasn't working, so what would it hurt? I grew up in a Catholic church where I never really got anything out of the masses I was forced to attend. It really seemed as though emphasis was placed on following rules over a relationship with Jesus when I was growing up. The worship services at the COE were laid back, each one having a theme. There would be a video and/or a song that we would listen to. Afterwards, we would discuss what it meant to us personally. It was the first time I felt comfortable enough to share my true feelings regarding God. I was in a judgment-free zone. The COE was a safe place with safe people. There wouldn't be anyone gossiping about me under the guise of 'special intentions', and I wasn't being tested on my ability to memorize scripture. It was freeing and led me to growing a genuine relationship with Jesus.

Patch is a member I'd sent to the COE the year before. I reached out to him and told him I was really enjoying the Sunday worship services. He was surprised they were still doing them. It turns out when he was there, they'd recently stopped bussing everyone who wanted to go over to an actual church due to Covid. Since they stopped going to the church, he decided he'd start holding Sunday Services at the center. It started out with only about eight people in attendance. It shouldn't surprise me because God always connects all the dots, but I was amazed that a guy I'd sent to the center started a worship service, that I would benefit from a year later.

I told my story to Pastor Tom, the guy who led the services. (He wasn't an actual pastor, but he had a strong faith and led our services, so that's what we all called him.) He found me later that day and told me that he would be graduating from the program soon. He needed someone to take over the Sunday worship service. He didn't know who it should be, until I told him about my connection with Patch, the guy who'd started it. He felt like it was confirmation that I should be the one to lead the service. I told him I was completely unqualified to lead, that surely someone else was more knowledgeable and equipped to take over his role.

I felt a pressing on my heart, and although I still didn't feel as though I was qualified, I agreed to take over his role. This also included leading the prayer at the graduations, which took place every Tuesday and Thursday. I did my best, and to this day, my faith is one of the most important things I took home from the center.

Jesus continued to pursue me, even when I was too proud to ask for help. Years ago, He met me on a park bench in South Lake Tahoe. Now He was meeting me where I'd hit rock bottom, alone in a treatment center in Maryland. It turns out Jesus was actually the rock at the bottom, steadying me when I was too broken to stand on my own.

On September 11th, we had a special service where Dr. Abby Morris gave a powerful speech. She spoke of Father Mychal Judge, who was the Chaplin for FDNY. He was killed in the 9/11 terrorist attack, but his words live on through a prayer that he wrote. She read us the prayer, and it really resonated in my soul. I refer to this prayer often and share it with people who are going through hard times. This is his prayer:

'Lord, take me where you want to go;

Let me meet who you want me to meet;

Tell me what you want me to say;

And keep me out of your way.'

-Father Mychal F. Judge

When I'm in my peer support role, I advocate for members to make sure they find a clinician that they click with. I found myself in a position where I had a clinician I didn't jive with at all. I knew it would make my recovery longer and harder, so I asked if they could switch me to someone else. They basically told me I was used to getting my way and a little adversity would be good for me. My fast track didn't exactly happen the way I planned it. We had to reschedule our Disney trip for two months later in December. I was obsessed with getting out in time to go on this trip, and when that didn't happen, I felt like I'd failed in some respect. I felt as though I had let down my family. Lauren was completely supportive, never placing any guilt or blame on me. She knew that Disney would still be there when we were ready. I still had some work to do.

We were allowed to have our phones for a short period of time every day except Tuesdays and Thursdays. One day when I had my phone out, I saw a wellness visit for my oldest son pop up. I called Lauren and asked her what the appointment was about. She told me our son had really been acting out, and she was hoping to get a referral to a good child therapist for him. I asked her when this started, and she told me it started after I had left. If you want to talk about a punch to the gut, this was it. I felt so much shame and guilt for contributing to my son's distress. We talked a lot about generational cycles and how we had the power to break the negative ones. I thought I'd broken some, but this news just made me feel as if the cycle was continuing, despite my best efforts to break it.

In my absence, the weight of the world was on Lauren to keep up with duties we usually shared. She had to take care of the boys, the house, the chores, all while working full-time. Both of our families stepped up and stood in the gap for us, helping with anything and everything. Lauren called our brother-in-law, Jack, who is a police officer, and asked him to come and take the guns I had in a safe at our house. I haven't seen them since Jack picked them up. Close friends of ours also showed up to help Lauren without being asked. A neighbor who knew I was gone took it upon himself to mow our grass. I cannot express how grateful I am to everyone who helped Lauren carry all of the weight in my absence. We have an amazing support system, and I may not vocalize it enough, but we couldn't have gotten through that season without them.

Part of the program at the COE forced me to take a deep dive into some of the trauma I'd endured in the past. Although I felt as though I had previously worked through a lot of it, I realized that while I'd touched on the events and worked through them, I never went all the way to the root of the problem. This allowed a lot of negative feelings to continue to rise to the surface. I dove all the way to the bottom and had a few moments of breakdowns that led to breakthroughs.

I recognized that I had some unresolved issues with my dad from childhood. I was encouraged to pick up the phone and have a hard conversation with him. We got along just fine, but in order for me to truly heal and move past some of my issues, I had to address this and talk to him. I'm so glad that I made that phone call. We had a really good conversation, and a lot of assumptions I'd made were cleared up for me. My dad genuinely felt bad that I was dealing with issues that stemmed back from my childhood. When we ended the conversation, my dad told me four words I'd been longing to hear: "I'm proud of you." I wish we would've had this conversation sooner, but better late than never.

I learned the power of forgiveness. I had to rid myself of the bitter poison I continued to carry and grant forgiveness to others. Not because they really deserved it, but because I deserved to be free of the toxic anger and resentment, once and for all. Growing in my relationship with Jesus, I knew that when we repent, He forgives us. But we're also called to forgive others, including ourselves. I started to forgive myself for burdens I've been walking with for years. This was probably the most difficult, but life altering, forgiveness I'd extended.

I ended up staying at the COE for a total of forty days. Towards the end I got discouraged, and my focus shifted on leaving instead of finishing out my recovery strong. Accountability is a big thing I was leaning into there, and they not so gently reminded me that I had to shift my focus and finish the good fight. After squeezing in about six-years' worth of therapy into forty days, I finally graduated the program. My flight was booked, and I was ecstatic to get home to my family. I assumed that, after my stay, I'd be boarding the plane back home completely healed. While I made a ton of progress, this wasn't the case. Contrary to common belief, my work on myself wasn't finished; I'd only begun.

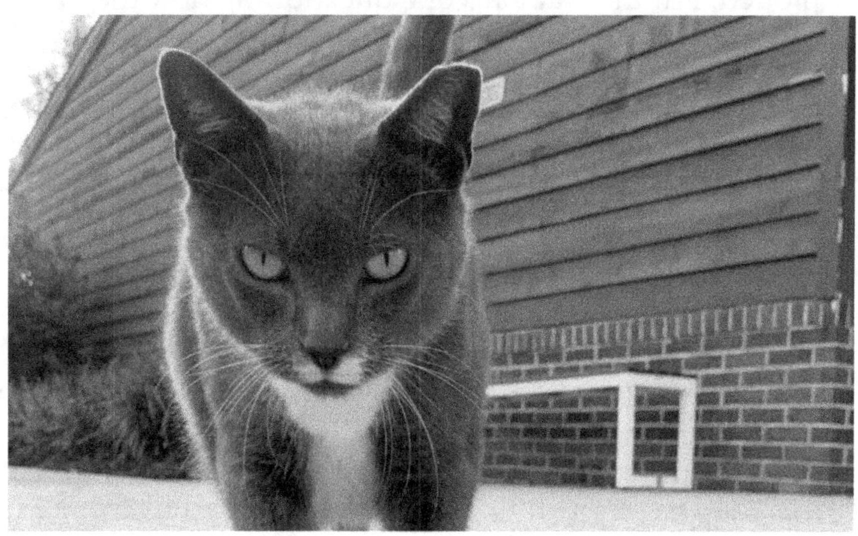

Tank the cat at the Center of Excellence

44 – BACK TO REALITY

"I did then what I knew how to do. Now that I know better, I do better."
-Maya Angelou

After a forty-day stay, I graduated from the Center of Excellence on September 29th. I was so happy to be heading home to my family. I was also a little nervous about life outside of the COE bubble.

I'd left home so abruptly I didn't really get a chance to explain to my close friends what had transpired. All they knew was that one day I hopped on a flight to Maryland for treatment; they didn't even know anything was wrong. After coming home, I invited my core group of friends over for a bonfire, where through crackling firewood and hazy smoke, I apologized for deceiving them. I thought lying to them would help preserve myself, but it only further isolated me from the people who genuinely care about my well-being. I explained to them when the chink in my armor occurred and when the steel shield imploded. I didn't want anyone questioning how they had missed the signs, or if they'd contributed to my unraveling. My friends met my confession and apology with grace, and were just happy that I was there and that I was okay. Although a lot of things were still up in the air, at least I knew that, moving forward, I had the support of an incredible group of friends.

The protocol after returning from the COE is to take two weeks off work and gradually reacclimate yourself back into your daily schedules and routines. I began going to the Kettering Intensive Outpatient Program (IOP) three days a week. I would return to work under restrictive duty for ninety days, per doctor's orders. I was originally assigned to report for duty at the headquarters, where my spiral really began. I knew that although I'd acquired great coping mechanisms, I wasn't ready to work there. I had to get the union president involved to have my restrictive duty assignment changed. My new assignment was working with my friend Steve, repairing radios. I was still in an extremely vulnerable state, and I often referred to Steve as my babysitter. I subtly changed my email signature from "Jim Burneka, Wellness Coordinator" to "Jim Burneka, Assistant to the Radio Repair Man." I had lost my title before I left for COE, but I would come to learn that my job or title didn't define who I was. Steve made sure to remind me that I didn't need a title; people were aware of who I was and what I've done, and that's enough.

I had to get my restrictive-duty paperwork signed by the deputy chief, but he wasn't there. Instead, I had to go to the assistant chief I'd had a huge falling out with. It was cordial but incredibly awkward for me. To ensure I would make it to my IOP, I'd start my day early. It was important to me to maintain the progress I'd made, but I still wasn't back to myself. I realized the city didn't consider what had happened to me an on-duty incident. With this epiphany, I knew there was no way I could return to the station, back to my old job. When it got close to the end of my ninety days, I submitted paperwork to the city requesting they extend my restrictive duty. The fire department was willing to work with me, seeing as I still had potential and they weren't ready to give up on me. However, the city didn't share the same sentiment and were quick to stamp my request with a hard no.

I'd been considering taking an early retirement through disability, but I felt as though I still had more to offer. The city made my decision for me, because I knew I couldn't go back into the literal and figurative fire that had burned me.

With the support of my clinicians and family, I began the process of filing for disability. I used all my sick leave and vacation time while waiting to see if the pension board would approve my disability claim.

No one knew my last day of restrictive duty would be my last day working for the City of Dayton Fire Department. There would be no fanfare, no hugs, no goodbyes. It was a far cry from the plan I'd laid out years ago. I only had three more years until I could officially retire. But neither of those facts mattered. The only one that did was that I mentally couldn't handle being back on the street. This would be the last day I shaved my face (except for an accidental shaving, but I still don't want to talk about that.) This would be the first day that I sought a medical marijuana dispensary and filled a prescription to help me sleep. I was certainly living a nightmare; this seemed to be my only shot at a brief opportunity to dream.

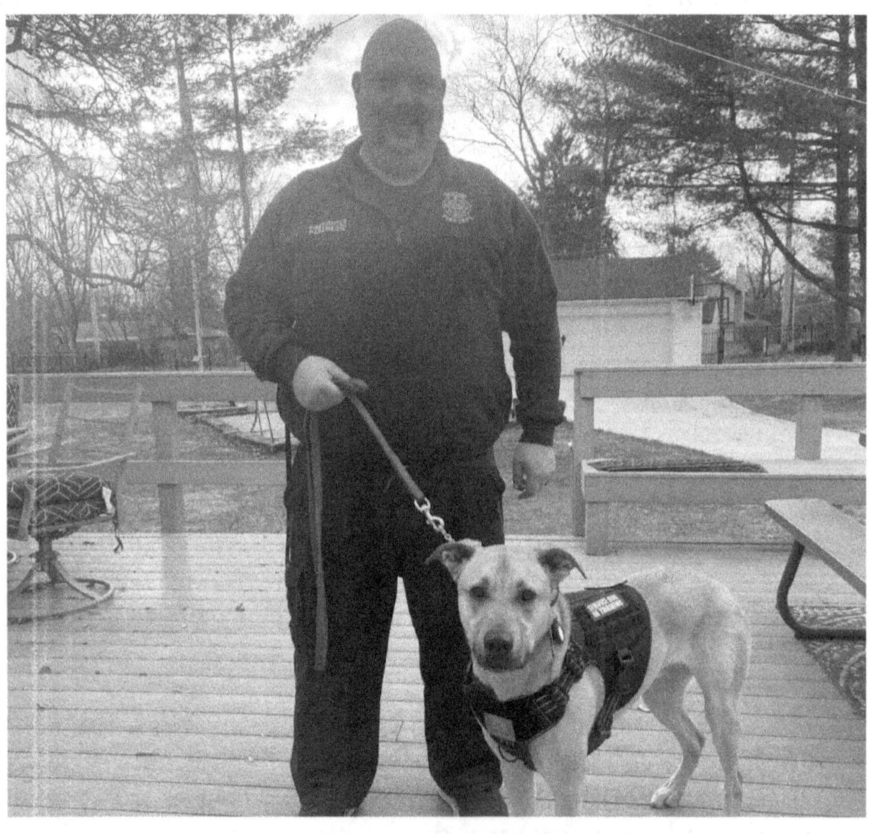

Last day I ever had this uniform on

45 – HAPPIEST PLACE ON EARTH

"When you wish upon a star,
Makes no difference who you are.
Anything your heart desires will come to you."
-Pinocchio

I'd experienced so much sadness and darkness, and I was looking forward to going to a place known for joyful experiences and memories. After saving and planning for a long time, my family was ecstatic to go to Disney World! We were originally supposed to go in October but ended up postponing the trip until December due to my unexpected stint at the Center of Excellence. We traded leaves, pumpkins, and spooky season for wreaths, bells, and Christmas magic.

After the tumultuous fall we had, our family desperately needed some fun and happy moments. We all got caught up in the Disney bubble, where the kids' excitement was contagious. Joyful Christmas carols floated throughout the attractions. There were massive Christmas trees throughout the parks, adorned in brightly colored ornaments and lights. The characters came to life, dancing past in parades with extravagant floats. The smell of freshly baked cookies and fudge filled the air. Every small detail was included in the extravagant decorations. Taking in all of the sights and sounds through the boys' eyes was an experience I will always treasure.

We quickly learned that Logan wasn't a fan of roller coasters, but Jameson couldn't get enough of them. Jameson and I rode the roller coasters, and Lauren and Logan went on some of the less intimidating rides.

We spent quite a bit of time in the new Star Wars area, Galaxy's Edge, and we built our own lightsabers and droids. We savored the delicious (but overpriced) food at the parks and fit in as many rides and attractions as we could.

During our trip I got a call from my attorney, saying they'd finally reached a settlement on my presumptive cancer claim. It felt as if someone had lifted a massive boulder off me. I was so relieved that I'd be getting back the time I'd taken off for my cancer surgery and recovery. This time would later be essential in bridging the gap between when my restrictive duty was up and when the pension board made a decision regarding my disability claim.

There were some moments where the crowds and overstimulation made me feel anxious, but I did my best to work through it for the sake of my family. I had high expectations for this trip, and Disney exceeded them. I hope when my boys look back, they think about the happy memories we created, versus my abrupt, forty-day absence. I don't know if there's enough fairy dust for that, but one can hope that lightsabers, cotton candy, and fireworks will always be a treasured memory they hold on to.

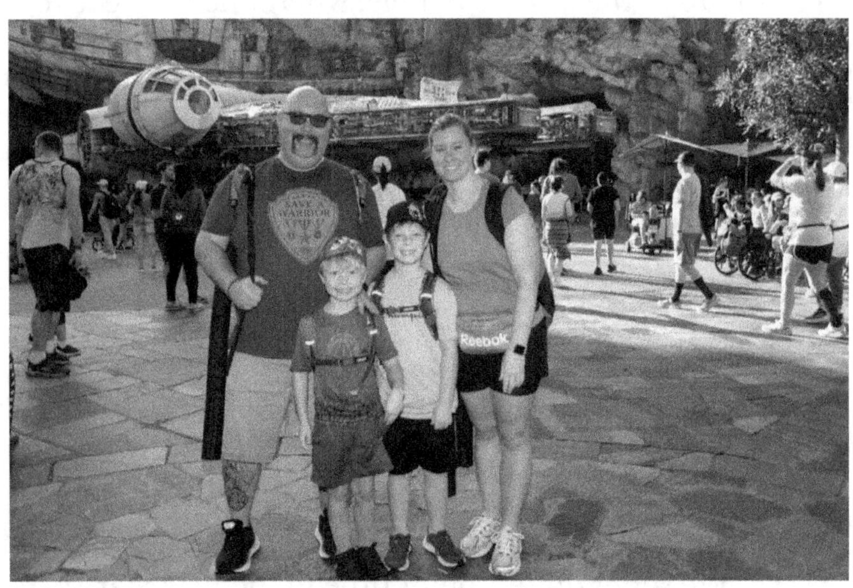

My family in front of the Millennium Falcon

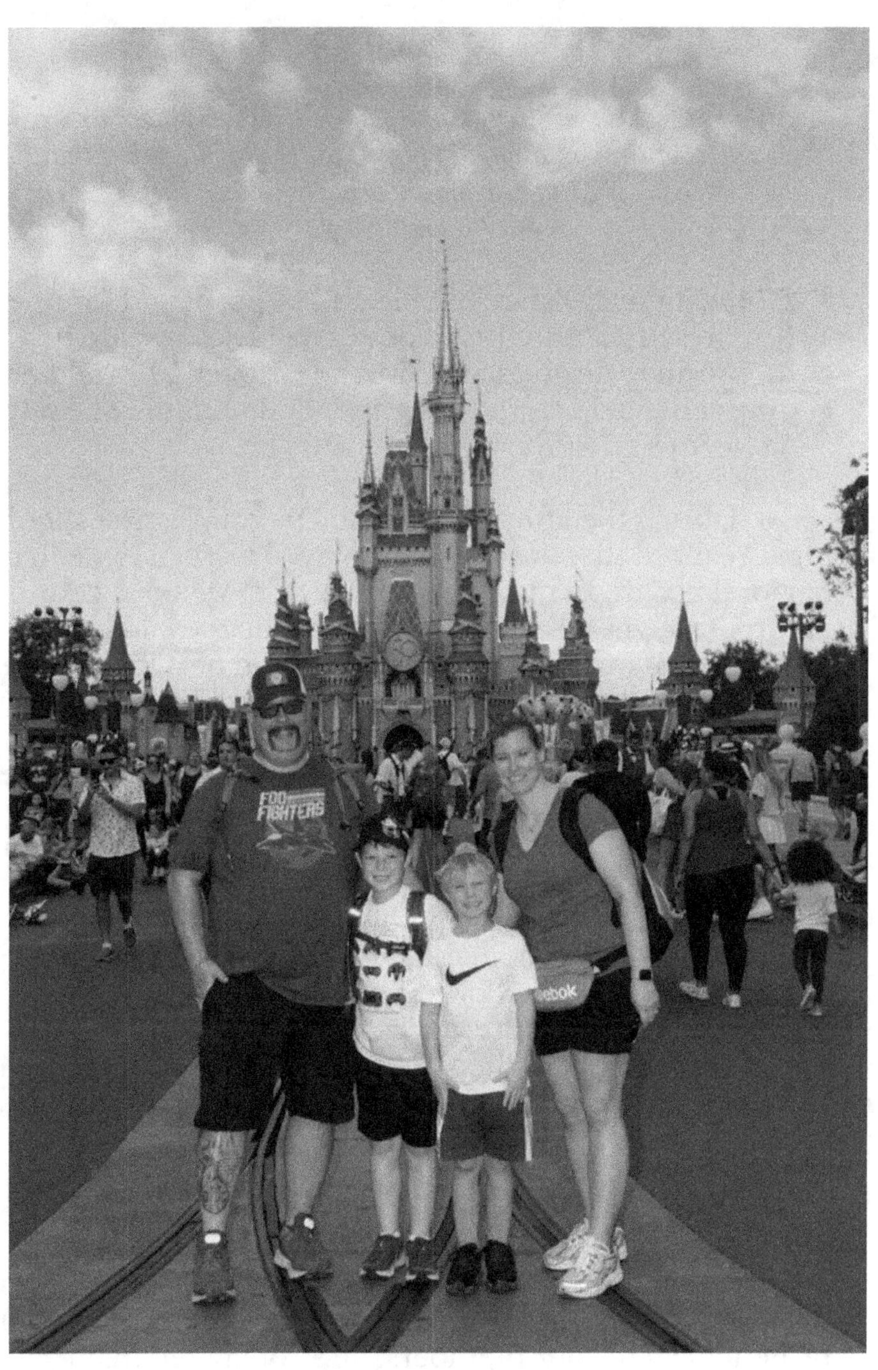

Magic Kingdom day

46 – BISHOP

"I have found that when you are deeply troubled, there are things you get from the silent devoted companionship of a dog that you can get from no other source."
-Doris Day

The joyous Disney bubble had popped, and I found myself back in the throes of trying to remain in a positive headspace. In just a few weeks, I would be getting some help from an eighty pound bundle of energy and sweetness. Let me back up a little bit.

During the aftermath of the Oregon District shooting, I realized that therapy dogs played a crucial role in behavioral health. In my role as the district wellness coordinator, I thought that having a therapy dog would be a great asset to our members. There would be a lot of benefits to having a therapy dog come to work with me. I knew firsthand that they helped ease anxiety, and who doesn't like having a dog around? I noticed when I went to stations or scenes, I'd start getting the guys talking and wondering who I was there to check in on. I thought having a therapy dog would allow me to access the firehouses and incident scenes without the guys thinking I was there to speak to one of them. I started investigating the process for getting a therapy dog. A friend of mine told me about an organization she saw at a conference called Dogs Helping Heroes. I reached out to them, inquiring about getting a therapy dog to partner with me in my wellness coordinator role.

While I was completing my treatment at the Center of Excellence (COE), a therapy/service dog came up in conversations I had there. I talked to a representative from the organization, and while he agreed a therapy dog might be beneficial for our members, he strongly felt that I needed to pursue getting a service dog for myself.

Let me clarify the difference between the two types of dogs. A *therapy dog* (what I was originally interested in) is used to bring joy to people other than their owners in a variety of places, such as hospitals, schools, or medical facilities. This dog works on a volunteer basis. They must have AKC Canine Good Citizen training, as well as certification from a therapy dog organization. A *service dog* works only for their owner. They help their owner navigate through everyday life. This dog must undergo extensive training in tasking and public access. They must pass a public access test in order to become registered as a service animal. Service dogs are permitted to go almost anywhere including restaurants and riding on planes. Therapy dogs are limited in where they can go and what they can do.

I didn't know if it would work out, but I thought I'd fill out an application for a dog while I was still at COE and see what happens. About two weeks after returning home from COE, I got a call from the Dogs Helping Heroes Organization, inviting my family to come out and do an interview. Although my wounds were still fresh, I had to go through and rehash all the things I'd been through that led me to possibly benefitting from a service dog. I got a phone call on the way home from one of the people in my interview and was told that the panel had unanimously voted I would be a good candidate for a service dog. In a way I was happy to hear that I would be getting a service dog. But another part of me wondered how messed up I must be for them to come to a decision so quickly and all in agreeance.

It took some time for them to find a dog that would be a good match for me. They were looking for a bigger dog that I could lean on to help me stand up. (I've had three surgeries on torn ligaments in my knees.) In December, we got a call to bring the family to meet the dog they thought would be a good match. We drove two and a half hours to meet the dog. I instantly liked him. He was a

Shepherd/Labrador mix, a good size, and had a sweet temperament. Lauren and the boys clicked with him too.

On December 16th, I went back and did my first training session with them. I brought home the perfect, though unexpected, Christmas present. When looking at names, I wanted his name to have a significant meaning. I landed on the name Bishop, which means guardian. Bishop-would be there to help guide me through this mess and protect me along the way.

I made the two-and-a-half-hour trek back and forth to meet his trainer eight times, but it was worth it. He is a strong, loyal, and sweet dog. Although he is a service dog, we've discovered that Bishop suffers from anxiety. We lean on each other to get us through anxious moments. It's funny that I initially started out looking for a dog to help other people and ended up with my own guardian. My journey has been a long and bumpy ride. I'm thankful that my detour included Bishop.

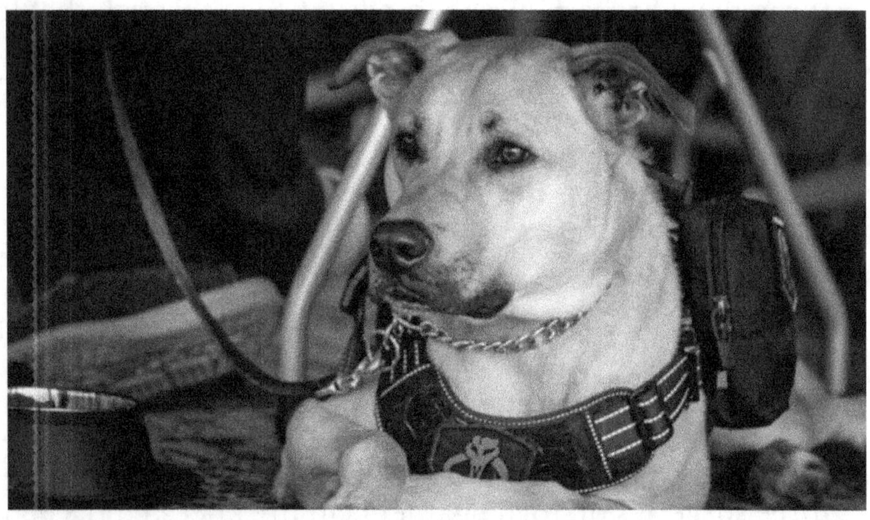

Bishop is a good boy.... yes, he is!

47 – HEALTHY HOBBIES

"People with many interests live, not only the longest, but the happiest."
-George Matthew Allen

I was keeping up with my clinician appointments and had my service dog, Bishop, to help me. However, when I was at the Center of Excellence, it became glaringly evident that I didn't have any real hobbies. Outside of my job and my family, I didn't have a healthy area to focus my energy on, or an escape that would allow me to decompress. My clinicians strongly advised me to seek a few new hobbies that would provide me a much-needed outlet. Since then, there are two hobbies I've picked up that I truly enjoy, and they help me to focus on something positive rather than allow anxiety or depression to take over.

The first hobby I've started is called pyrography. (I know, cue the jokes. I can't get away from burning things.) Basically, this is woodburning. I like to create various pieces of artwork using this method and typically gift my creations to friends. I've made a wide variety of signs and quotes. I set up a work area in my garage to do this. It's a great release and allows me to be laser-focused on something that's positive.

I have a hundred-disc Rowe jukebox in my garage, and I always play this when I'm doing pyrography, or if I just want to lighten my mood. We all have phones that have the capability to play any song at any given moment, but there's just something special about a jukebox. It's cathartic flipping through the various albums, choosing an artist and which songs I want to hear. There are songs to accompany any mood. It's easy to get lost in artwork while listening to the music float out of the speakers. There's something magical and nostalgic about that jukebox; it's truly healing for me.

Another hobby I picked up is Frisbee golf. It gets me out of the house and in nature, and it's a fun method of decompressing. I have some good friends that I routinely play with, and it's been really good for me. This reminds me of a funny story that some of you will appreciate. When I was a kid, there was a local record store that also sold some toys and disc golf items. I went in and referred to it as "Frisbee golf" instead of "disc golf." The guy working got mad and told me, "Frisbee is a trademark of Wham-o," in the voice of the comic-book guy from the *Simpsons*.

Whether you're in the midst of a mental health battle or not, you should acquire some hobbies that capture your interest. Finding a hobby you enjoy will provide a number of health benefits to you mentally, emotionally, as well as physically. It's never too late to start something new!

It's been gratifying exploring new interests. Along with new hobbies, I was getting ready to expand upon my current level of teaching experience, and attempt to check off a bucket list item in the process. I'm learning that we need to quit limiting ourselves, because we are capable of achieving far more than we could ever imagine.

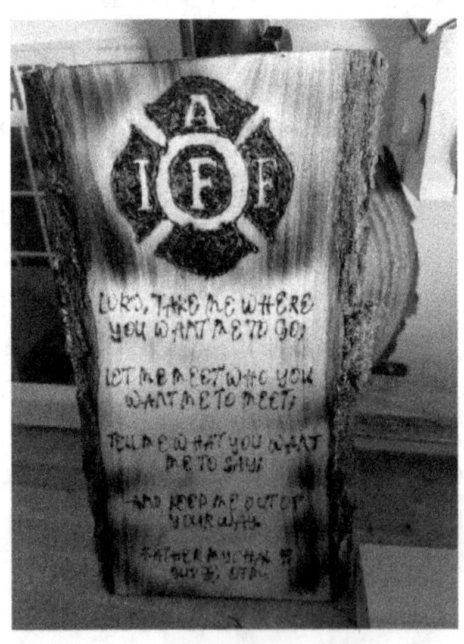

48 – CONCERTS AND EVENTS

*"There is some good in this world, Mr. Frodo, and it's worth
fighting for."*
-Samwise Gamgee

I found some activities that gave me a healthy outlet, but one thing that has always been cathartic to me is music. Music has always given me an easy escape. Anyone who knows me knows that I'm an avid concert goer. I love nothing more than traveling to a concert, relaxing, and having a good time with Lauren and my friends. It isn't just concerts that I love attending, I also love most sporting events and comedy shows. I couldn't even count the number of these events I've gone to in the past.

I remember after the Oregon District shooting, Hootie and the Blowfish were reuniting in Indianapolis. I bought tickets to the concert, thinking it would be the perfect escape from the aftermath of the mass shooting. Lauren and I traveled there, anticipating a fun night away. It was great until Darius Rucker (the lead singer) started talking about the Oregon District shooting and honoring the victims. It was a natural thing to do, but it totally ruined the rest of the night for me. The videos in my head from that night began playing on loop, and I couldn't turn them off. After unexpectedly being triggered, I told Lauren we needed to leave. I felt bad that I ruined her night away, but I needed to get out of there.

My anxiety and hypervigilance continued to grow from there. Any time I was in a crowded area, I began worrying about who else was in the crowd, and my mind automatically began playing out worst-case scenarios. My distrust for the general public grew to the point that I looked at *everyone* as a potential threat. I couldn't get out of my head with this. I stopped going to these events altogether for a while. They were no longer enjoyable and had actually become extremely stressful for me.

I was given a prescription of medical marijuana, and I've found it takes the edge off just enough that I can go to concerts and events, and not be miserable the entire time. It helps turn down the volume in my mind, where screams of what could go wrong reverberate between my ears. I know it isn't a permanent solution, but for now it's a crutch I use to help me overcome the anxiety I experience in large crowds.

If you or a loved one are experiencing debilitating anxiety or hypervigilance, it could very well be a symptom of a much bigger issue. I know these behaviors may seem rare if you're experiencing them, but believe me when I tell you this is a very common problem. Please seek the medical opinion of a clinician. There are various methods for treating anxiety that may work for you. No one should have to give up something they love due to mental health issues that can be treated!

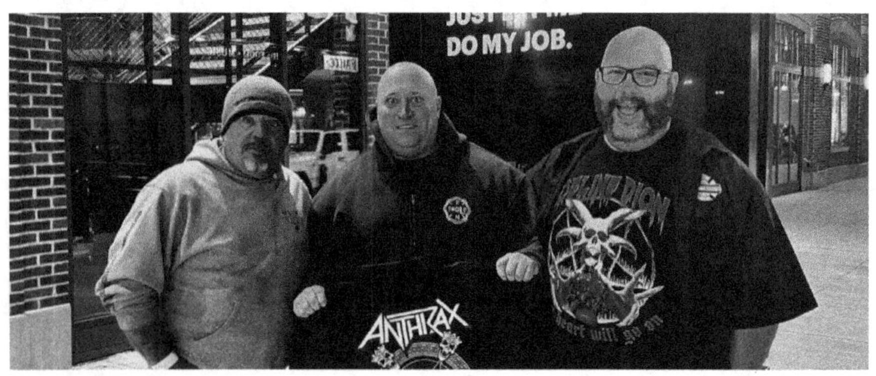

Yep, I wore a Celine Dion shirt to an Anthrax show

49 – FDIC

I was happy with the progress that I'd made thus far, and I didn't want to stop attempting to achieve my goals. One goal that felt out of reach for a long time was to teach a class at the Fire Department Instructors Conference (FDIC). This is the largest firefighter conference in North America. The conference is held annually in Indianapolis, Indiana. Typically, about 35,000 people from around the world attend this conference. It is a top-notch conference, and the who's who for teaching. I submitted proposals for years trying to teach a cancer prevention/awareness class, but never received approval to teach at the conference.

I took a different approach in 2022 and submitted a new proposal to teach a class called "How to Create and Enhance Your Fire Department's Health and Wellness Program." Are you ready for the irony here? I found out that my proposal was accepted during my stint at the Center of Excellence. After years of trying, I was finally approved to teach a health and wellness class—while I was at a health and wellness rehabilitation center. The irony was uncanny. I called Lauren and we both had to laugh about it. What I had originally thought was irony at its finest actually worked out for great teaching material for my class. My original plan was very textbook heavy, with a lot of important information. After my stay at COE, I was able to incorporate real-life scenarios into my class. I taught them valuable information, but I also used my own circumstances to teach how easy a slip turns into a slide, and that *everyone* has a tipping point. I wanted them to understand how imperative it is to seek help before reaching their tipping point. I know from my own experiences that often times people attend a class covering a topic they are struggling with. I was done with my act and had taken off my mask before going to Maryland. I owned my problems and where they led me. In doing so, I found that vulnerability breeds vulnerability. A lot of people were receptive to what I taught and opened up about their own personal struggles. I actually shared this speech that I wrote during my stay at the COE with the attendees:

I received a lot of positive feedback from the people who attended my class. I was feeling pretty good about how the conference went. I checked out of the hotel on a high note, only to find the valet guy waiting for me outside with my truck. My truck, which had a massive dent and scrape on it that wasn't there when I dropped it off. He told me one of their drivers had an incident and accidentally ran my truck into a pole in their parking garage. Fortunately, my truck was still drivable. I made the two-hour trek home from FDIC, thankful for the opportunity I'd been given. The partially wrecked truck couldn't put a damper on my feelings of accomplishment, and I finally checked teaching at FDIC off the bucket list.

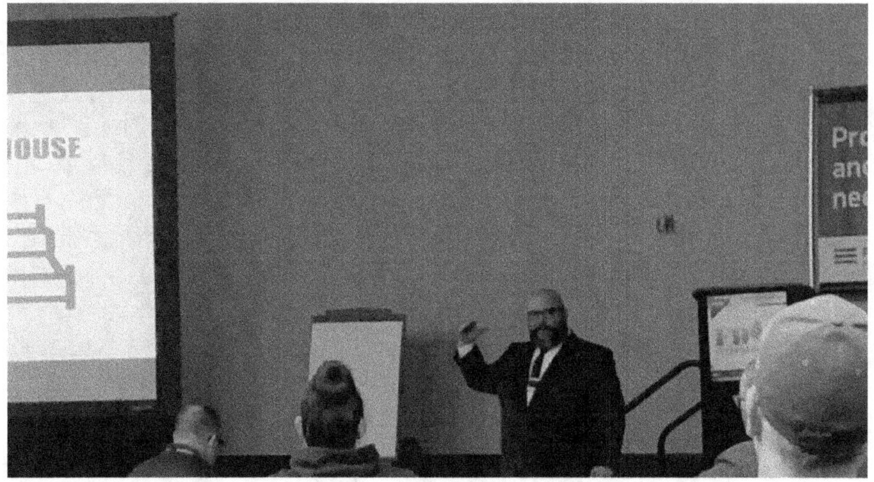

Finally teaching at FDIC

50 – WORTH A SHOT (SGB)

"You miss 100% of the shots you don't take."
-Wayne Gretzky

Coming off the heels of a weekend at FDIC, I was feeling motivated to optimize any tool available that could potentially increase my overall health. A friend of mine who was in Chicago reached out to me and told me that he'd just received an injection that drastically decreased his post-traumatic stress (PTS) symptoms. He instantly felt lighter and had less anxiety after receiving the shot. He was really excited about this breakthrough he had. I hadn't heard of this treatment, and the same day, a different friend of mine also mentioned the treatment out of the blue in a conversation. I was intrigued and wanted to learn more about this shot.

After doing a little research, I learned that the stellate ganglion is a collection of sympathetic nerves that are located in the front of your neck. They are basically the routing center in the nervous system for the fight or flight response. The stellate ganglion is what seems to control the activation of the amygdala, the fear center of the brain. The shot my friends were telling me about is called a stellate ganglion block (SGB). It is essentially a chemical injected into that collection of nerves, which can reset the sympathetic nervous system to its pre-trauma state. While the shot is not a cure for PTS, it can help control the symptoms. A lot of people feel more relaxed, experience less anxiety, and are able to sleep immediately after receiving the injection. Doctors use this shot for soldiers in the military to help decrease chronic pain. They noticed a side effect to the shot was that it seemed to calm the mental state of some of the soldiers. The results can last weeks to years, differing in each person.

The shot is not effective in everyone; it has about a 75-80% success rate in decreasing PTS symptoms. Those were pretty good statistics, and I knew I wanted to try this shot. Best case scenario, it relieved my anxiety, insomnia, and eliminated the horror movies that played in my mind each night. Worst case scenario was that it wouldn't work, but there was no risk in trying.

I made the trip to Chicago, hopeful that this shot could help alleviate some of the symptoms I was experiencing. Unfortunately for me, the shot was not effective. I landed within the small 20% of people that couldn't feel a difference after receiving the injection. I was disappointed, but I knew going into the procedure that it wasn't guaranteed to work.

I would recommend this option for someone who has been suffering from symptoms of PTS. There is no shame in trying a treatment which can help alleviate some of the symptoms. It's worth giving it a shot (pun intended). There are several treatment options that are beginning to gain traction, such as microdosing, ketamine, and the SGB injection. Microdosing is taking a very small dose of a psychedelic to help relieve symptoms without experiencing the negative side effects of the drugs. Ketamine is an anesthetic used in treatment-resistant or very severe depression. All of these treatment options should be done under the care of a trusted physician. They won't work for everyone, but it won't hurt to research the treatment options that are out there and to try what you feel comfortable with. Healing is a process, and there's no shame in utilizing these tools to help you throughout your healing journey. In the following chapter, I'll delve into my journey of trying to find the correct hormone balance with the help of injections.

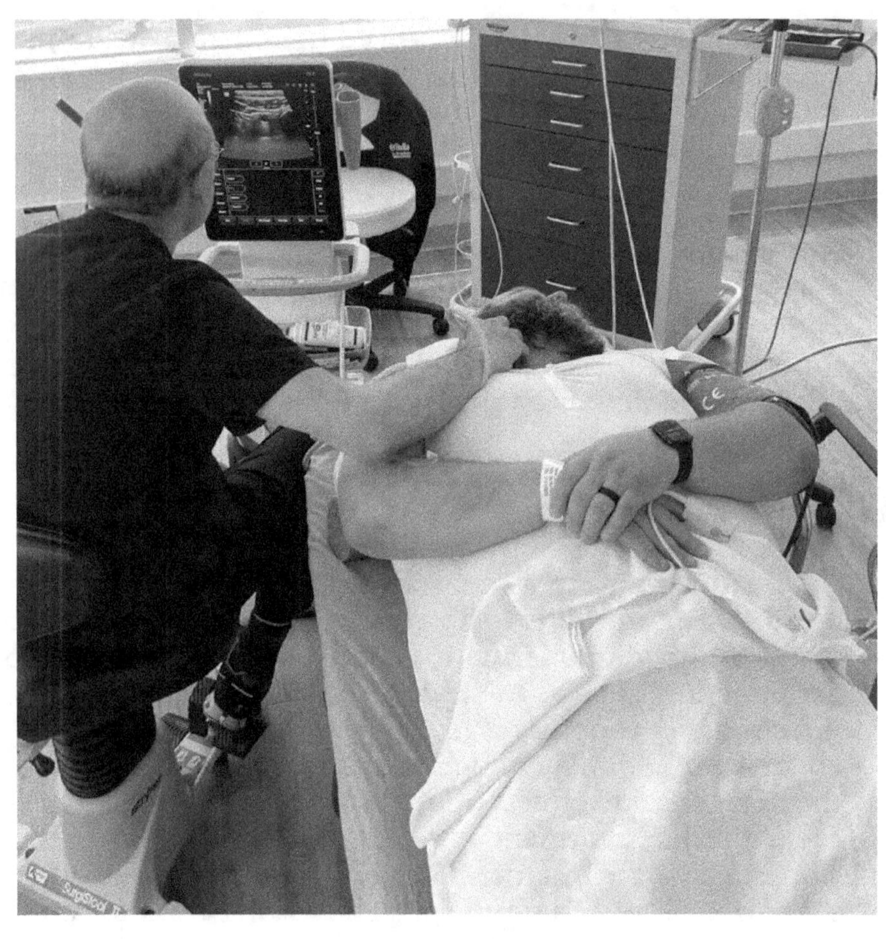

Dr. Lipov searching for the injection site

51 – MAN, I FEEL LIKE A WOMAN

"Let's go, girls!"
– Shania Twain

There's a common misconception that firefighters lie around the firehouse all day, occasionally going on runs to rescue lost cats that are stuck in trees. The reality is that our job wreaks havoc on our bodies. The majority of calls we respond to happen between the hours of 6 p.m. and 6 a.m. Being woken up out of a dead sleep to an alarm ramps up adrenaline and cortisol levels. Repeat this cycle several times throughout the night, and your body's natural rhythms are all out of whack.

The body's main stress hormone is called cortisol. It communicates to the brain to help control mood or fear. When the body experiences stress, (physical or emotional), the cortisol levels rise, creating a fight or flight response. The constant stress firefighters have on the job results in increased cortisol levels, which in turn, decreases testosterone levels. For example, if firefighters are fighting a fire for longer than twenty minutes, their heart rates will be elevated, which increases the cortisol levels. When the body experiences prolonged stress, sometimes the testosterone production stops to allow the body's fight or flight response to kick in.

About six or seven years ago, I noticed that I was feeling drained all of the time. Even if I had a great night's sleep and a relaxing day, I felt exhausted. Several guys I knew had these symptoms, and it was due to low testosterone levels. One appointment with an endocrinologist later, and sure enough, my testosterone levels were low. I started taking a supplement to help increase my levels, but when those didn't work, I had to resort to getting weekly testosterone shots. I've been receiving these shots for years now.

After my stay at the COE, I noticed that I was extremely emotional. I've never really been one to cry, but all of the sudden I would feel the urge to cry out of the blue. It was baffling behavior for me. I was telling my friend Matt about this, and he asked me if I was taking an estrogen blocker along with the testosterone shots I'd been getting. In all of the years I'd been getting the testosterone shots, I'd never received an estrogen blocker. He told me that was a huge problem, because those shots increase estrogen as well as testosterone. Matt encouraged me to find a new endocrinologist who could properly regulate my hormone levels.

I went back to my doctor and had him test my estrogen levels. A healthy range level of estrogen in a man is between sixty and one hundred ninety. My estrogen level was at 435.3—off the charts. I couldn't help but wonder if this absurd chemical imbalance had contributed to the mental health struggles I'd been going through. It was no wonder I felt so emotional all of the time.

I'm not telling you this because I think you have an interest in my hormone levels. I'm including this because, due to the nature of the job, it's common for firefighters to experience low testosterone levels. Please, learn from my mistake and make sure that if you're taking testosterone supplements, you are ALSO taking an estrogen blocker!

"Helping others is the way we help ourselves."
-Oprah Winfrey

When trying to heal from any mental injury, I believe it's imperative to utilize all of the tools and resources available. I've talked about how imperative it is to see a clinician to receive help processing the trauma we encounter, and thought I would offer some perspective from my personal experience with clinicians.

My first experience with a clinician was when Lauren and I went to my Employee Assistance Program (EAP). I went there seeking help because I was experiencing anger issues. I think this is a valuable program the city has, but my personal experience is that the clinicians aren't specifically trained to help first responders with the level of trauma they experience.

From there I met Alison, who's the founder of Pinpoint Behavioral Health Center. Her husband is a firefighter, and they taught a class together at the union hall. She caught my attention during this class when she mentioned firefighters getting emotional over things that typically would not make a person feel emotional. I was experiencing that very sentiment and was intrigued with how she could help me overcome my heightened emotions. I worked with her for a little bit, but we both realized that we'd be working together through peer support, and thought it would be best if we maintained a professional relationship versus a clinician/patient relationship. She put me in touch with a clinician who works for her named Sabrina. I've been seeing Sabrina consistently for the past four or five years now. She walked me through my first EMDR session, and I have also done horse therapy with her. I enjoyed doing equestrian therapy. Horses are so big and powerful, but they're also really in tune with human emotions. They can sense when you aren't calm, and some will be standoffish with you until you maintain a calmer disposition. Sabrina has played a huge role in my healing journey.

When I was at the Center of Excellence, Lauren and I did virtual couples' therapy. We both got a lot out of those sessions and wanted to continue them once I came back home. We started working with a therapist who was a nice man, but we just didn't click with him. I didn't feel as though I could be myself and would hold back during our sessions. This definitely hindered our progress. We cut ties with him and found the current therapist we work with, Roxanna. She's located in California, so our visits are virtual, but they're still very effective. Lauren and I both trust her and enjoy our sessions with her.

I understand that seeking a clinician can be a daunting task for someone unfamiliar with therapy. Knowing where to start can be overwhelming, especially if you're mentally struggling. If you think that you could benefit from therapy (honestly, we all can), a good place to begin is to ask if your department has a peer support team, and if such a team exists, speak to someone on the team. They can act as a liaison and help connect you to an already vetted therapist who specializes in what you need help with. If the station you work for doesn't have a peer support team in place, you can look online for resources that can point you in the right direction. For example, here in Dayton, I currently keep up our local Dayton peer support page. You can take a look at: **https://www.136peersupport.org**. On a state level, there should be resources available to you as well, such as this site from the Ohio Association of Professional Firefighters (OAPFF): **https://firefightermentalhealth.org**.

If you cannot find anything in your area, you can always start at **https://www.psychologytoday.com/us**. This is a website you can use to narrow down the search for a therapist that is close to where you live, specializes in the area you need help with, and accepts the type of insurance you carry. If you find someone that is a great fit but they aren't covered by your insurance, sometimes you can apply for a grant or scholarship and get your sessions covered through one of those. Do not automatically give up if insurance is an issue!

If you are a first responder going in blind as you seek a therapist, the International Association of Firefighters has an excellent page of questions you can ask potential clinicians. There are seven questions that they recommend you asking. They are as follows:

1. Do you have experience working with firefighters or other emergency responders, including EMS, police, or military populations?

2. What evidence-based practices do you use to treat post-traumatic stress disorder, depression, anxiety, and co-occurring substance abuse? Do you assign homework?

3. How many sessions does it typically take for you to complete your initial assessment?

4. Do you offer appointments within 24 hours or access to an on-call clinician?

5. If an individual has a psychiatric emergency and needs inpatient care, what facility or hospital do you refer to?

6. Do you work closely with a prescriber for individuals who need medication?

7. Would you be willing to participate in experiential training to gain a better understanding of the daily experiences of the fire service professional?

Questions are found at: **https://www.iaff.org/wp-content/uploads/2019/04/Finding_the_right_Clinician_Flyer_2018.pdf**

Remember, if you're a first responder, the criteria that a clinician must meet will look a little different for you versus someone that doesn't frequently experience trauma. It may take trying out a few different clinicians before finding one that is a great fit, and there is nothing wrong with that! Don't get discouraged in your search for a good match, because the right therapist is out there, and you will gain so many benefits from working with them. I have experienced this, and it can be frustrating, but it's absolutely worth the effort!

Personally speaking, I don't foresee the day that I'm not working with a clinician. They play such a major role in my mental health and healing journey. I encourage you to find a clinician you click with and continue working with them. It's an investment in yourself that's well worth the time and money. The clinicians I work with have immensely helped me sort through difficult subjects, including my path forward on my healing journey. Ultimately, they helped me come to the only conclusion that made sense in allowing me to heal and experience a healthy future with my family.

53 – RETIREMENT

"For I know the plans I have for you, declares the Lord, plans to prosper you and not to harm you, plans to give you hope and a future."
-Jeremiah 29:11

When I was at the Center of Excellence, I had to re-hash my story to at least four different clinicians (all separately). All four of them asked me how much longer I had until I could retire, and if retirement was a serious option. I went into the Fire Academy right out of high school, so I only had about three more years until I could retire. In the grand scheme of things, three years is nothing. My clinicians and I realized that in my case, three years would seem like a lifetime.

After working with me for some time, the clinicians brought up disability as an option. I happened to have a virtual mediation with my attorney and the City of Dayton regarding my presumptive cancer claim. I had asked my attorney if disability was a viable option for me. She told me that she wasn't sure, and that in her experience filing for disability was a very long and drawn-out process.

I brought it up to Lauren, and we even had conversations about it with the clinician during our virtual counseling sessions. The clinicians at COE strongly felt that I needed to get out of the environment that had caused me so much turmoil and truly work on getting healthy again. Lauren and I talked in depth about what that would look like for us. We also talked about my fear of being harshly judged by others.

I knew that what the clinicians were saying made sense, but I also knew that it's looked down upon to go out on disability. I was so close to the finish line; I didn't want to prematurely quit.

Throughout my career, there had been several times that I stood up to the City of Dayton and really became a thorn in their side. One example of this was going to the press about the hypocrisy they showed in the way they treat employees who've been diagnosed with occupational cancer. I was certain that because I was an outspoken advocate for the members of Dayton Fire, the city was not going to go out of their way to accommodate me in any fashion.

As I mentioned previously, the fire department recognized my merit and was willing to work with me. The city, however, was not. They denied my request to extend my restrictive duty, and pretty much made the decision for me to pursue disability.

The process to apply for disability was lengthy and complicated. I had to gather all the injuries and illnesses I had sustained while on the job. There were a lot, including three ACL reconstructive surgeries and cancer. I had to see two separate doctors in Columbus, a psychologist and a general practitioner, to evaluate my physical and mental health. Once they completed their evaluations, I could apply for disability.

The pension board sent me to three of their doctors to complete further evaluations. I had to see a psychologist, a doctor to evaluate my physical health, as well as an occupational doctor. I had to wait months for the pension board to meet and review my application. During the time I was waiting, I ran out of sick leave and vacation time. For about a month, we were stretched thin living on only Lauren's paycheck. It was stressful, but I felt a peace knowing that God had a plan for me that was bigger than my own, and His purpose would prevail.

On June 21st, my attorney called and told me that my disability claim had been approved. I felt so much relief, like I'd finally broken free of the chains that had held me captive.

I had to let my station know that the pension board approved my disability, and I'd officially be retiring. I scheduled an exit interview for Friday, June 23rd. I'd also have to turn in my gear at the training center. My exit interview was with the district chief that long ago refused to allow me to bring any members to the union hall during the Workman incident. He made my role as a peer support coordinator extremely difficult. There was a point in time that a mutual friend of ours offered to sit down with us and mediate a conversation so that we could bury the hatchet. I was willing, but the district chief declined. I knew this interview was going to probably be unlike any interview he had ever conducted. During my interview we both aired out our grievances towards one another and admitted we both had regrets on how we'd handled past situations. We genuinely apologized and forgave each other. A grudge that had formed over fifteen years ago was finally broken. We hugged each other at the end, and I believe healing had taken place in both of us. I really wish we hadn't waited so long to have this peace with each other, but I'm glad that we at least found a place of grace and forgiveness.

I drove away and took a picture of the training center in my rearview mirror. I posted the picture on my social media, with the caption, "Across the tracks. What a long, strange trip it's been." It was two tiny sentences, but the implications were huge. The easiest way to sum up how I felt in the moment was with a nice quote from Jerry Garcia and the Grateful Dead.

A lot of my close friends started asking me if I was going to have a retirement party. I told them I didn't have any intention of throwing a party. While I felt relief about retiring, I also felt a lot of guilt, shame, and embarrassment. Retiring early through disability is generally not celebrated. If anything, it is frowned upon. It didn't feel as though I'd reached the end of an era; it felt as though I'd come up short on a lifelong goal.

My true friends urged me to have a little party, so I planned one at the Dublin Pub. Whereas these events are typically open to anyone, I only invited a select list of people that I knew were supportive of me. We displayed some photos of me throughout the twenty-two years of my career as a firefighter and paramedic. In a plot twist, I invited the chief that I'd had so many problems with but reconciled, and to everyone's amazement, he showed up. I realized that while I may never celebrate the reasons that led me to take an early retirement, I should celebrate what I've accomplished throughout my career. As a member of peer support and as wellness coordinator, there are a lot of stories I cannot tell due to confidentiality, but I knew where I had made a difference. I knew the lives I'd saved, and the lives that I had positively impacted.

I no longer run into burning buildings to fight against blazing flames; but I'm now fighting to reignite the flame that has gone dim within myself. I am asking God to take the black ash that has accumulated in my soul and bring goodness and beauty from it. Some of you might view my retirement as me giving up. I'm going to tell you that you are wrong; I have just started fighting.

When we first started writing this book, my retirement was going to be the end of the story. After all, the story outlines the joys and heartbreak I've experienced throughout my job. Now, after settling into the idea of retirement and gaining my bearings, I realized that while retirement from my job was the end of a chapter, it's not the end of my story.

I can't tell you exactly where my story is going, because I'm not the author of life plans. Instead of fearing the fact that I'm not solely in control of my own life, I'm embracing the fact that God is. Just when I felt as if my life no longer had purpose, I felt the words "the comeback" permeate my soul. This new chapter is not a sad tale of an early retirement, but an exciting adventure of making a comeback that I never thought would be possible. Does it look the way I thought it would? Of course not. But I've learned that life rarely looks the way we think it should. I'm excited to continue to heal and help others along the way. This road that I'm walking feels narrow and I can't see very far ahead. After blindly walking through unbearable *pain*, I'm now confidently stepping into my *purpose*. I know in the midst of pain, it doesn't seem possible, but I promise there is purpose on the other side of pain.

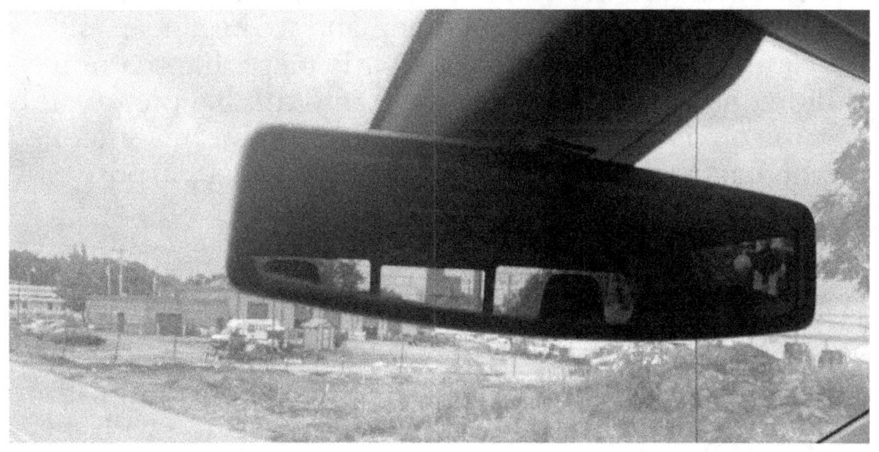

Across the tracks and in my rearview

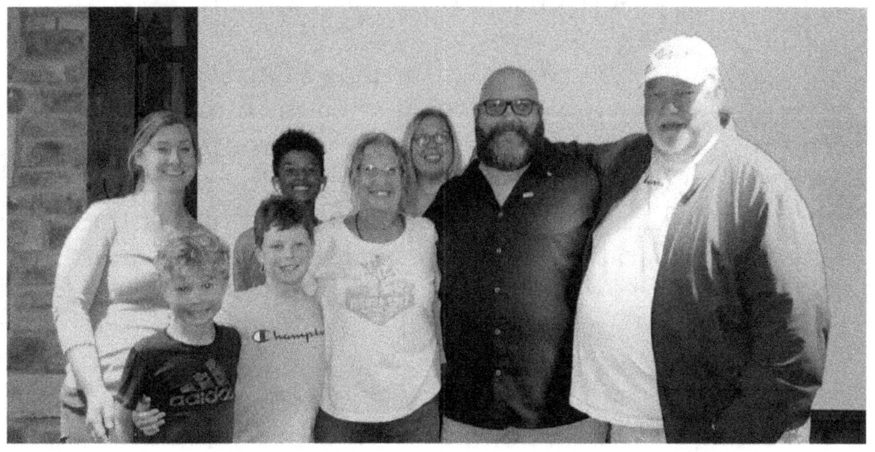

Some of my family members at my retirement party

54 – EPILOGUE

"Not all those who wander are lost."
J.R.R Tolkien

I used to think that I had a lot of bad luck. Crappy things would happen to me out of nowhere, and I would go from one frustration to the next. As I sat down and told my story to my sister, all of the puzzle pieces started to come together, and we began seeing a beautiful picture. Each jagged little piece that seemingly didn't have a place in my life fit into this big picture. It became obvious that I wasn't merely a victim or someone who had a lot of bad luck. Each piece had a purpose and prepared me for the next part of my life.

For example, if I didn't help Sean with Gavin's fundraiser, I wouldn't have met the founder of the Firefighter Cancer Support Network (FCSN). If I hadn't met him, I wouldn't have been able to hold a position within their organization. If I didn't lose my position with the FCSN, I wouldn't have started my own company, the Firefighter Cancer Consultants. I can confidently say that these events in my life weren't coincidences; they were all appointed by God, all a part of a bigger plan.

When you are going through a hard season, don't give up on your life and assume that nothing will come from these tough seasons. I am living proof that you can go from feeling utterly hopeless to finding purpose in your life. What I deemed as some kind of punishment was actually preparation. For a while, I felt like an exile from the very world I'd immersed myself in for over two decades. But was I an exile, or had I finally found the path that would lead to my calling?

The heartbeat behind this book is to help others avoid making the mistakes I made. Please, seek help *as soon* as you are starting to feel depressed or anxious. There are no trauma trophies given out for people who never seek help; nothing positive will come from silently suffering (trust me on this).

Each act of betrayal, depression, anxiety, and trauma I experienced were all sewn into my story, combining into an invisible thread within my body. I have come to realize the thread that I thought unraveled me, actually connected my broken pieces. The thread not only connected my shattered pieces, but stitched together my gaping wounds, finally allowing me to heal from the trauma I have endured. I will inevitably bear some scars, but I'll never cover them in shame.

For, by the grace of God, I have overcome Tuesday.

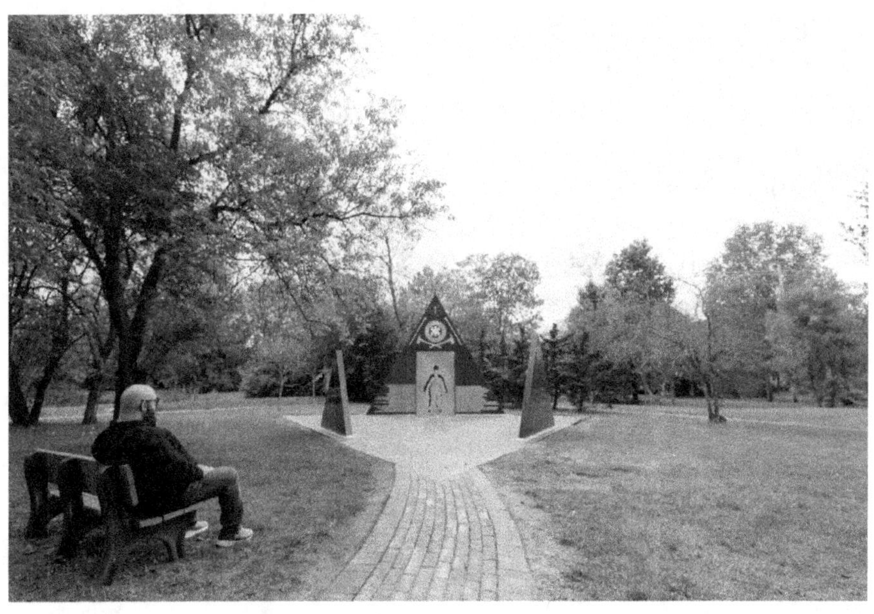

Sitting in front of the Miami Valley Firefighter EMS Memorial in Centerville Ohio

988 Suicide & Crisis Lifeline - https://988lifeline.org

Ace Quiz- Source - https://cls.unc.edu/wp-content/uploads/sites/3019/2016/08/From-ACES-TOOHIGH-ACES-and-Resilience-questions.pdf

Behind the Shield Podcast - https://www.jamesgeering.com

Brothers Helping Brothers - https://www.brothershelpingbrothers.org

Center of Excellence - https://www.iaffrecoverycenter.com

Dayton Firefighters Local 136 Peer Support - https://www.136peersupport.org

Dogs Helping Heroes - https://www.dogshelpingheroes.org

Dr. Donnie Hutchinson - https://donniehutchinson.com

Firefighter Cancer Consultants - https://firefightercancerconsultants.com

Firefighter Cancer Support Network - https://firefightercancersupport.org

Fire Department Instructors Conference (FDIC) - https://www.fdic.com

First Responders Bridge Retreat - https://firstrespondersbridge.org

International Association of Firefighters(IAFF) Fallen Firefighter Memorial - https://www.iaff.org/fffm23/

International Association of Firefighters Questions for Clinicians (IAFF) - https://www.iaff.org/wp-content/uploads/2019/04/Finding_the_right_Clinician_Flyer_2018.pdf

Ohio ASSIST - https://statepatrol.ohio.gov/about-us/ohio-assist/

Ohio Association of Professional Firefighters- https://firefightermentalhealth.org

Opportunities for Ohioans with Disabilities - https://ood.ohio.gov/home

Pinpoint Behavioral Health Center - https://www.pinpointbhs.com

Post-Traumatic Stress Disorder Information - https://www.mayoclinic.org/diseases-conditions/post-traumatic-stress-disorder/symptoms-causes/syc-20355967

Psychology Today- https://www.psychologytoday.com/us

Save a Warrior (SAW) - https://saveawarrior.org

Sleep Apnea Information - https://my.clevelandclinic.org/health/diseases/8718-sleep-apnea

The Chip Terry Fund - https://www.thechipterryfund.org

56 – BOOK RECOMMENDATIONS

Check out these books if you enjoyed ours:

Challenges of the Firefighter Marriage –
Mike & Anne Gagliano

Create Your Own Light – Travis Howze

Cornerstones of Leadership – Frank Leeb

Emotional Survival for Law Enforcement –
Dr. Kevin Gilmartin

Exposure – Rob Bilott

Firefighter Functional Fitness –
Dan Kerrigan & Jim Moss

Granite Mountain – Brendan McDonough

Lead With Balance – Dr. Donnie Hutchinson

One More Light – James Geering

Relentless Courage – Michael Sugrue & Shauna Springer

Taking the Cape Off – Patrick J. Kenny

Tattoos and Trauma – Dr. David Griffin

Was it Irony or Was it God? – Lisa J. Taylor

When the Calls Stop – Dr. Mynda Ohs

Why We Sleep – Matthew Walker

Thanks for reading! Please add a short review on Amazon and let us know what you think!

To stay up to date on different topics that we are interested in and or writing about, feel free to check out our link trees. This also has our contact information if you have any questions.

https://linktr.ee/jimburnekajr

https://linktr.ee/hilaryhawkins

www.ingramcontent.com/pod-product-compliance
Lightning Source LLC
Chambersburg PA
CBHW071412150726
48000CB00001B/286